New Organs Within Us

EXPERIMENTAL FUTURES
Technological Lives, Scientific Arts, Anthropological Voices
A series edited by Michael M. J. Fischer and Joseph Dumit

NEW ORGANS WITHIN US

Transplants and the Moral Economy

ASLIHAN SANAL

DUKE UNIVERSITY PRESS *Durham & London* 2011

© 2011 Duke University Press
All rights reserved
Printed in the United States of America
on acid-free paper ∞
Designed by Jennifer Hill
Typeset in Arno Pro by Achorn International, Inc.

Library of Congress Cataloging-in-Publication Data
appear on the last printed page of this book.

For my family

Der Mensch kennt nur sich selbst, insofern er die Welt kennt, die er nur in sich und sich nur in ihr gewahr wird. Jeder neue Gegenstand, wohl beschaut, schließt ein neues Organ in uns auf.

A man knows himself insofar as he knows the world, which he perceives only within himself, and himself only within it. Every new object, properly examined, reveals a new organ within us.

JOHANN WOLFGANG VON GOETHE,
Poetische Werke, Band 1–16

CONTENTS

THE ACCURATE NATURE OF THINGS

She could be herself, by herself. And that was what now she often felt the need of—to think; well, not even to think. To be silent; to be alone. All the being and the doing, expansive, glittering, vocal, evaporated; and one shrunk, with a sense of solemnity, to being oneself, a wedge-shaped core of darkness, something invisible to others. . . . When life sank down for a moment, the range of experience seemed limitless. . . . Beneath it is all dark, it is all spreading, it is unfathomably deep; but now and again, we rise to the surface and that is what you see us by.

VIRGINIA WOOLF, *To the Lighthouse*

Zehra was used to living in a dream world in her solitary life, but bodily changes had destroyed the calmness of her inner world, replacing it with doubt and the fear of surveillance—as if people could see through her now, as if they watched her dreams, read her thoughts, observed her movements. Her life first on the dialysis machine and then with a transplanted kidney awakened things inside her that were hard to accept and even harder to reveal.

Zehra did not know when it had begun, but it was long before 2001, when she, at the age of twenty-seven, received her father's kidney at a public hospital's transplantation unit in Istanbul. Despite her knowledge that change was normal and came naturally, she still had a hard time grasping her new biological tie to her father in the form of her transplanted kidney, her new dependency on the hospital's rules, routines, and prescriptions, and her relationships with the doctors and other patients there. If everything went well and her body did not reject her

father's kidney, maybe she could once again believe that what had constituted her past, her memories, her daily life—what constituted herself—
was based not on lies, but on truth: that her father was really her biological
father, bolstered by the fact that the tissue type test proved him to be a possible kidney donor, and that her religion, the minority Alevi denomination
of Islam, was not the religion of infidels as she had been told during one of
the shuttle rides to dialysis, but did lead to the true path to paradise.

Zehra's kidneys had failed in 1997. At the time she lived in a town in the
Black Sea region. Her initial symptoms were weakness, a draining fatigue,
swelling, and a pain that crept slowly up her back, symptoms that resembled those of her uncle, who had suffered renal failure years before and had
died. The unfortunate uncle had traveled to Istanbul very often for treatment and was on and off dialysis. Just as everyone thought he was getting
better, one day on his way to Istanbul on the bus he died. Mainly because
her parents understood the seriousness of the illness, when Zehra began to
have similar symptoms, they decided to take her to a hospital in Istanbul to
have her examined by good physicians. That is how she left her village, her
family, and the green landscape of her home.

At the hospital she felt she had to endure a lot. She found it an unpleasant place: many of the doctors and nurses were overworked, and they rarely
treated her nicely. Unlike all the usual things that happen to a person, the
beginning of her diagnosis and treatment marked her life like no other experience. During her first visit in the hospital, she had to stay there for two
weeks as "important doctors" in white coats ran a variety of tests on her.
She began crying when they told her that she would have to start dialysis.
There was nothing she could do. They opened "a hole" or fistula (Turkish, *fiskür*) on her left arm to which the dialysis equipment could be connected. She had hoped for a long-term treatment that would restore life to
her own kidney. She did not want to be connected to a machine for the rest
of her life—that didn't even seem like a treatment. But the physicians gave
her no other choice.

She began spending three hours a day at the dialysis unit, attached to
the machine. After the treatment she would throw up for the rest of the day,
her blood pressure would be unbalanced, she would suffer joint, ankle, and
neck pain, and she would be unable to walk properly. Painkillers were only
a temporary solution. In a short while, she began feeling as if her body were
no longer her own, as if the body she had once known as hers was slowly

being replaced with something else during the dialysis cycles, as fluids entered her body and her own blood was circulated out before her eyes.

Dreams became her reality during the dialysis, as she would try sleeping to avoid interacting with her fellow patients. Often she sunk into half-sleep and had a recurring dream. In her dream, she was *makinada* (at the machine, or attached to the machine) undergoing dialysis. Suddenly the IVs would come out and she could not fix them. But she would remain physically connected to the machine somehow and could not move regardless. She would look around desperately for a nurse who could help her put the needles back into her arm. Blood would pour from her arm, and while the sight would shock her, she would feel no pain. Then she would wake up and everything would be normal. Once, as she sunk into sleep to have this same dream, it materialized: she woke up to see the needles dangling from her arm. Unlike her dream she was not bleeding.

Her body changed, her arm and her blood vessels swelled, and these changes bore others. Around the same time, as she began observing physical changes, she began to see things differently. It was as if she had been given new eyes and new insight. She recognized new ties to the dialysis patients she shared the treatment room with—her "new family." She had never been very talkative—she moved and socialized shyly because of a limp that was the result of a childhood fever. But with this new family she had to be more engaging than with her own family, since they could not read into her silences and reserved moods. Her new family bonded over the machines and conversed about them. Zehra preferred sleeping, but when the knot of her headscarf pushed uncomfortably against her neck as she lay back against the pillow and made her unable to drift off, she had to turn her head to the side toward her neighbor, who then talked to her even though she was not eager to talk to anyone in the room. Her fellow patient was an elderly man she referred to as the *dede*, which is colloquial for grandfather. And despite her desire for privacy, she did not want to be disrespectful to this man. If she could escape him, she would sink into dreams, but otherwise she listened.

On one of those days at the machine, an incredible thing happened. Zehra had turned her head to the side because her headscarf was hurting her neck when she saw that the *dede* had changed appearance: his nose had changed shape and was now arched just like hers. His hands looked like her hands, his thumb had the same unusual flat and narrow shape as hers, and there was henna all over his palms. Seeing the henna, the curved nose, and the narrow, flat thumb, she suddenly recognized this man: he must be her relative. Had she not realized before how similar she and the *dede* were to one another, and how different she was from her own family? At that moment she found herself in another reality, perhaps frightfully becoming aware of what Jacques Lacan called "the Real," that which is beyond the faculty of comprehension.[1] She must have been related to this man, and not to her own parents. It was not the first time she had questioned her ties to her family. With her bad foot and her dependence on the dialysis machine, she was not like any of her immediate family members. Her similarity to the *dede*, however, was remarkable and significant. This awareness shook her belief in her roots. She kept this experience a secret from the doctors to avoid being laughed at or put on psychiatric medication. But as her life sank down for a moment, it marked for her the beginning of a new set of feelings and possibilities for experiences, which seemed endless, fragmented, and frightening.

Other changes followed. Zehra would see the doctors' skin and hair change color as they approached her. One doctor looked dark-skinned and dark-eyed from afar, but when he came closer his appearance morphed by the second—his hair turned gray and his eyes became green, as if he were physically transforming as he moved. Another time she saw a group of doctors who were all dressed in black, an unusual color for the hospital. She was sure she saw these things change, but she was not positive about the cause: was it the light or was it her? If it was the light, merely an optical illusion, then she was just misinterpreting nature. But if people and objects really were changing shape to reveal their true appearance to her and she all of a sudden had insight into the miracles of a world unseen by others, then she could not talk about it. This kind of experience could not be shared with doctors or her family; it was personal. She started wondering how her experience of the world had become so deep and abnormal, if she was losing her sanity while trying to maintain her physical health, or if the world was indeed revealing its secrets to her. She had a deep desire to know the truth, for she had felt the dark shadow of death at her bedside a few times already. What kind of a truth was her experience revealing? Was she changing, in her body, her skin, her self? Or was it the people around her? She could not but wonder as she neared her death.

One day, after treatments in the hospital for a year and a half, Zehra fainted during dialysis and was taken to the emergency room. She changed her dialysis unit for a change in her environment. In time, away from the tensions of the hospital, she was able to return to her old job, helping one of her uncles at his small neighborhood grocery store a few days a week. Zehra used to work at textile sweatshops to contribute to her family's household income. After her kidneys failed, her uncle's shop became a very convenient place to work; it was close to her new home in Istanbul and she could have flexible hours. Her illness kept her busy, as she had to follow a strict diet, suffered from low blood pressure, and was too tired to do anything after dialysis. Basic daily routines began occupying all of her life and her body, to the point that she began to feel depressed. Amid the strains of her illness, it was very convenient to be able to work in a family environment.

Away from the hospital, at the small private dialysis unit, her life had a different quality. She would take a private shuttle to and from the dialysis three times a week, chatting with other patients from the center along the way. Everyone in the shuttle suffered from the same illness, the same pain, the same social death and isolation. During the hours they spent sitting in Istanbul's dense, dusty traffic, they often talked about religious and spiritual issues: death and the afterlife, and how Sunnis, the religious majority in Turkey, would go to heaven and, some suggested, how the minority Alevis would suffer in purgatory. Zehra was made uncomfortable by these talks.

"I was not so sure what we were . . . so I asked my mother if we were Alevi." At twenty-seven Zehra began to question her religious background for the first time in her life. Her mother confirmed that they were. This made Zehra even more distressed about her own afterlife. If the Sunni women on the shuttle were right, if their ways of practicing Islam were correct, then Alevis' practices, rituals, gatherings, songs, prayers, and all of her family's traditions that gave meaning to her existence in this world were wrong. That would mean she and all the other Alevis would go to hell. Why, she wondered, would so many people choose the wrong way? The Alevis were about 25 percent of Turkey's Muslim population, outnumbered by the Sunni population, which accounted for almost all of the remaining 75 percent. The shuttle conversations troubled Zehra. Life at home was as usual with everyone bringing a little to share at the end of the day. To them, "the end" was merely a romantic word in a prayer or a song. But Zehra felt her own end was nearing, and no one else understood her. Thursday evenings her family usually gathered at home to read and discuss verses from the Berat Kitabı (a prayer book), and then sing *ilahi*s (chants) together. One week, exhausted by dialysis, she was too tired to join the prayers. This sparked an argument with her brother, which soon escalated. She began telling her family how she felt about being an Alevi and how she was worried about being on the wrong path. None of them were dying, but she—she would soon have to face the truth. What if she burned in hell? Who had the right to say what is true anyway? Angered by Zehra's doubt, her brother became very angry and yelled at her, "*Sen bizden değilsin!*" (You are not one of us!)[2]

Zehra felt dismissed, unwanted, undesired. At the same time, however, this was exactly what she had suspected. She must never have been one of them (her immediate family as well as her community). If she were, she would have been as healthy as they were, but with her lameness and poor constitution she had been different from the very beginning, and now her kidney was failing as well. She might be related to the *dede* instead—he looked like her and he suffered like her. With her home and community environment destabilized like this, her notion of the afterlife became even more confused, and she started reading popular religious and psychology books in the hopes of escaping the possibility of purgatory. She wanted to become a part of the community that would wake up on the Day of Judgment and walk the narrow path between this world and the next with ease, but she knew she did not have much time left.

A few days before her transplant surgery, another thing had happened that confirmed that her end was near. She was undergoing treatment at the dialysis center when she saw a dark shade approaching the left-hand side of her bed. She recognized it at once as Azrail, the angel that came to collect souls: it was her death. "There he stood," she told me, gesturing weakly with her left arm, staring into emptiness. I looked at the spot she was pointing to by her bedside. "I saw him come close, and I could not breathe, but then he left," she said. As she was telling me about her moment, death had joined us, and I was struck by how beings from invisible realms made themselves visible to the eager heart.

When first I met Zehra and spent two long days chatting with her in the hospital, she had just received a kidney transplant from her father. Her already frail body was further weakened; she had a gentle, tired look in her eyes. She shared with me what she seemed to have kept secret from others, especially her suspicion that her father was not her "real"—biological—father. Despite the success of the operation, she remained unsure of it. *"Eğer bedenim böbreği atarsa bileceğim"* (I will know if my body rejects the kidney), she told me, meaning that she would know he was not her real father. All of the tests had gone smoothly, and tissue and blood types had matched. On account of this matching biology, she thought, he must be her father. Yet, her recent experiences had raised profound questions about the truth of her biological constitution and her kinship ties as well as her religion. Zehra believed for this reason that only her body could give her the ultimate answer, tell her who she and her family really were, tell her what the truth was and if she would see Azrail again soon.

Death was near and the unusual modifications of her reality were a sign of its presence. With her "new family" in the dialysis unit, Zehra had shared an invalid life of machine dependency, but also a life of dreams, visions, and illusions that revealed unexpected truths. In the dialysis room, she and patients like her talked about family, school, flirtations, kidney thefts, the "organ mafia," where to find transplant kidneys, and the rich and their good fortune—in short, everything one would talk about with close friends and family. Even though they had not known each other for long, they felt intimately connected through the machines and their failing bodies in a new biomedical world.

After the operation, Zehra was released from the hospital to join her normal family life at home, and since she no longer had to leave for dialysis, she could spend more time working at her uncle's market. But she was still uncertain of her father's blood tie with her, and though she had been cured of her ailing kidney, she continued to have other unusual experiences: she felt like people on television were looking at her, watching her, or speaking to her from behind the screen. When she watched the news, she felt certain that the anchorwoman was looking her in the eye as if she were talking directly to her. Her family was unusually kind to her now. Even her sisters, with whom she had had good and bad days in the past, treated her like someone else. They were too considerate, or too nice, or too quiet. All around her, she felt increasing attention directed to her presence. She had become the center of a world that surveilled her. Her paranoia grew. She felt changed: for as long as she could remember, she had been invisible to people, to her family and even to colleagues—except for when her boss at a sweatshop made indecent romantic overtures toward her. This she remembered very well; she had rebuffed him and quit the job. But other than this incident, she thought no one ever noticed her. After the transplant though, she had become the center of a world she could not recognize.

Zehra's condition was aggravated at the time of her transplant; it was as if she remained frozen and the world changed and morphed observing her. Could she feel, think, and move? Was she suddenly recognizing the truth of the world as it really was? Had she discovered that that truth was a far less tangible object than she had thought before?

The man Zehra called the *dede* was more to her than an elder. *Dede* is colloquial for grandfather, but the term also has another meaning. *Dedeler* (the plural of *dede*) are seen as saints and for this reason they are the leaders of Alevi religious and community life—they are believed to know the path to the truth and are chosen to lead people to righteous action. Their presence and knowledge allows traditions to take their course. As an individual, the *dede* does not have healing powers or conduct exorcisms, but he is believed to be nearer to God than other people.[3] Nevertheless, his role is utterly social, concerned with uniting the community, opening and closing the *cems* (religious gatherings) with poems, singing the *ilahi*s (chants), and playing the *saz* (an instrument resembling a lute). The *dede* speaks about sociopolitical issues, educates the youth about Alevi culture, and makes peace among rivals.[4] But in addition to this important worldly political authority, he is also regarded as half-sacred.[5] The *dede* represents the incarnation of knowledge, which is not solely divine, but mainly stemming from his life experience and wisdom. It is in the domain of the *knowable* and the common sense, along with the aesthetics of the *unknowable* divine, that the *dede* dominates the politics of everyday life among the Alevi.[6]

What then could the morphing *dede* have meant to Zehra's becoming? To Zehra her ill elderly neighbor from the dialysis unit, whom she thought of as the *dede*, might have possessed qualities of a respectable person because of his seniority. At the same time, with the use of the word *dede*, saintly qualities of a community leader might have been transported into this man's appearance so much so that in time he could morph to become like her to show her where she belonged: to the dialysis family but also to the Alevi community. As a *dede* on dialysis, he was half-sacred but also half-machine. As a morphing *dede*, he was half-divine but also half-her. The *dede*'s change in appearance to resemble Zehra was a comforting sign of the transformation of her own kinship ties: she did not get entirely detached from how she was bound to the world; she was linked to the other dialysis patients but also remained in the community she had belonged to all along.

In time, other seemingly unrelated things became significant to the meaning of her life. It was almost as if physicians' unfamiliar medical knowledge had found its way into her insides through the hole in her arm causing faces to morph, diffusing their world into her being, not only giving her clear signs of danger but also making her the center of an unbearable, oppressive, and technologically induced attention.[7] Bound to the dialysis machine, Zehra had been without will or desire and began becoming possessed by things and forces that she had never recognized in her inner life before. She could not place herself in the world any longer, or her relationship to God, which was determined by the fate of her community's beliefs. Her experience of the supernatural had a stronger affect than the scientific fact represented in her knowledge of the biological—the tissue match with her father. Yet, with the boundaries of things shaken, she hardly understood where things belonged. Facts mattered less in a world distorted such as hers. Experience—no matter how odd and unusual—became the elementary form of her relationship with herself, not only with others, and the path to true knowledge.

For me, Zehra's crossing over represents the point where the boundary between fact and fiction, wish and oppression, truth and reality, and dream-state and nature-state vanished. For Freud, *the fact that people could dream* helps them invent worlds of personal significance and opened possibilities for further imaginaries. In the dream-state, nature re-organized itself. In his *Interpretation of Dreams*, looking into his own dreams and life experiences, Freud suggested that wish fulfillment was the main drive behind dreams, that dream life operated like a kind of psychic energy—in his interpretation, a libidinal energy—the underlying element upon which real-life experiences were built. In the invention of technoscientific imaginaries such as Zehra's, biological knowledge takes over the authority of the intuitive and the desirable, chaining the person to a former lifeworld, from which she can hardly escape. As the binary oppositions inherent in the dream-versus nature-states vanish, comprehension is taken over by an altogether new sense that literally perceives social life as one's own body.

In between the ailing body and her *unknowable* future, Zehra's *akl-ı selim* (common sense) had built herself a life-world, a new space, a parallel universe. In turn, she felt, this world began watching her. The rapid emotional and moral changes that came with her body at the machine, and afterward the incorporation of the new kidney, allowed her to enter another reality that made invisible and unthinkable forms appear. Thus speakers from television screens started talking to her, sending her signs that she could interpret to find her own way. This unusual care was overwhelming. It was a loving surveillance, a tyranny of affection, a reading of the world through mimicry, gestures, symbols, and signs. She could follow changes in an abstract and unique world where she was the heroine. She could read the world like she never had before. And just like that, a savage mind arose from beneath her perception of daily events—in between others' worlds but now wholly in them. She had morphed.

WHAT MAKES THE WORLD OUR OWN

As he moves about within his mental and historical framework, man takes along with him all the positions he has already occupied, and all those he will occupy. He is everywhere at one and the same time; he is a crowd surging forward abreast, and constantly recapitulating the whole series of previous stages. For we live in several worlds, each truer than the one it encloses, and itself false in relation to the one which encompasses it. Some are known to us through action; some lived through in thought; but the seeming contradiction resulting from their coexistence is solved in the obligation we feel to grant a meaning to the nearest and to deny any furthest away; whereas the truth lies in a progressive dilating of the meaning, but in reverse order, up to the point at which it explodes.

CLAUDE LÉVI-STRAUSS, *Tristes Tropiques*

Like Zehra, many transplant patients spoke to me of a changed sense of being as they talked about their "new life." They were becoming familiar with distant worlds condensed in a biomedical universe under construction. There, medical professionals were trying to draw a fine line in their decisions on what they believed to be culturally *desirable* or *impossible*—and in the process determining the sensitivities of the biomedical field.

In this book, I write about inner changes as we try to handle the emotional affects of biomedical technologies that can have the effect of making life seem as though it were a psychotic experience in need of repair and reconstruction. As the anthropologist Claude Lévi-Strauss so vividly describes, we humans live in many different worlds at once, and we deploy techniques—rites, rituals, and discourses—in a dialectical fashion to give meaning to our individual lives. Normally we follow the "natural" connections of these worlds; we weave continuity in our lives by granting meaning to the nearest contexts and denying meaning to those furthest away. But if the opposite happens, we experience it as unusual, or as Lévi-Strauss puts it, unnerving shifting of grounds of meaning as in an explosion of truth. I have come to think of the transplant experience in terms of such a "truth explosion," a detachment from previous reality resembling psychosis. Yet this truth explosion is different: it is initiated by all that technology represents and it happens when one has to relate to distant realities through affect triggered and elicited by transplant technologies.

This book begins with organ transplant patients in Istanbul such as Zehra, but it doesn't stay in Istanbul or Turkey or with only kidneys and their transplantation. It follows the connections of meaning as Lévi-Strauss suggests. From the point of experience, transplant patients, their doctors, their families, and the various others whose roles come into play could be anywhere as my ethnography entails stories related to Europe, Russia, India, Israel, Iraq, the United States, and even Nigeria. This, in a way, is one of the promises of ethnography: that deeply observed particular cases can throw light on processes more generally connecting our individual experiences to those of others, making them meaningful. Likewise, the stories I tell are about anxieties and hope as well as resources and connections. They are about the "Other" sides of new "life-saving" biotechnologies, the troubled human sides. I speak of shifting legal categories known as white, gray, and black markets; the public and social democratic mode of political economies versus the private and neoliberal mode; the stratified access to health for rich and poor citizens in rich and poor countries; the demands of family; and especially the contested meanings of life in this world and the next. The particularities of these meanings are deeply personal, cultural, historical, and social, and their translation through ethnographic detailing is how we can come to an understanding of the emerging worlds around us and come to terms with their ethical and moral challenges.

Over the years, I have met many physicians and patients who spoke of change to me: transplant patients' experiences—the bodies they have made their own—were posing a most unusual relationship with nature compared to the ways they previously related to their lifeworlds. When patients were diagnosed with renal failure and lost kidneys, they would become part of a high-tech biomedical world that hosted intense medical practices, a complex economy, reincarnated human organs, and transnational boundaries. All these separate worlds seemed to fill their inner void while they mourned the loss of an organ.

Because of their physical condition, transplant patients were forced to live in several interconnected worlds, which gave birth in them to a new inner knowledge. Goethe, like Lévi-Strauss, captured this experience, writing that "a man knows himself insofar as he knows the world, which he perceives only within himself, and himself only within it. Every new object, properly examined, reveals a new organ within us."[1]

Inside us are people, relations, worlds encountered. Articulating these, Freud also thought, were organs, veins, bones. Like Goethe, he believed that the world outside had its imprints inside. More specifically Freud was interested in the part that had been marked upon the biological—in those parts of the somatic that were rooted in the psychogenic and the social. Both Goethe and Freud observed the spaces and gaps of loss. That was precisely where the transplant discourse for my interviewees with transplant patients, doctors, brokers, television journalists, and others also began.

In his classic essay, "Mourning and Melancholia," Freud distinguished between mourning and melancholia, which he thought were two processes, one complete, the other incomplete, and both branching out from the same root cause of the *loss* of a loved object. If the loss was mourned and replaced by another object, in time the person would recover. If the person was not able to replace the loss, then she or he would project feelings for that object upon his or her own ego and sink into melancholy amid self-pity and narcissism. To me, Freud's analysis was inspiring mainly for two reasons. First, he talked about the *loss of an object*, which actually was the loss of a relationship. Second, he talked about its character. These were "internal objects" that constituted our inner lives; they had been made personal; they had been internalized. They existed in the external world as well as within the walls of our own little inner universes, just as Goethe had said so poetically. We related to the world through these objects we had made our own; our relationships to them constituted the meaning of our lives.

In Turkish, there is a technical term for internalization: *içselleştirme*. But there is also a traditional word that I think is more fitting in the context of my own work with transplant patients: *benimseme*, a word that originates in the noun *ben* (I) and turns it into a verb, *benimsemek* (I-ing). *Benimseme* means becoming familiar or feeling at ease with something by making it one's own. It also means internalization in a less technical and more colloquial way. It is a powerful word used to describe how the self, *ben*, or the ego, can incorporate things, turn the world into its own territory and extend a feeling of relatedness into the world. It entails positive feelings of ease and comfort with the relationship and its object. When I alternate the terms internalization, or making one's own through out this book, I actually refer to all that *benimseme* entails: the ways technology is made personal, affect is interpreted, and people can begin to feel at ease with themselves despite initial troubles.

Also following the tradition of "object relations" that stems from Freud's essay "Mourning and Melancholia," I began viewing internal objects as things that we learn to relate to upon certain preconditions and promises fished out and reorganized from the domain that Jacques Lacan calls "the Real," that is, a realm of diachronic discourse beyond the individual's faculty of comprehension or consciousness.[2] In this case, I write about technological objects, products of scientific research. In my research, what made these technological objects particularly distinct and evocative[3] was that they had lost either their social or their biological wholeness; they had less life, or they were *life-less*. A living-related organ donor, the donor body of a suicide, the cadaver of an insane person, or the skeleton of a foreigner: these were human bodies, dead or alive, commodified to be used for medical ends, as I discuss in part 2. I thought of these *life-less* objects' place within the transplant experience in two stages of *benimseme*. To begin, I tried to understand how the loss of personhood affected its relation to its biological host (and vice versa), and how this new "altered relation" could be utilized culturally as a *life-less* epistemic quality so that these objects could be used for medical purposes. In the context of my own work among transplant patients and physicians, the first stage took place in the medical setting and involved regulations, rites, and rituals. The second stage was how this experience made itself a room in peoples' inner worlds.

In its local Turkish context, I thought of the medical setting as a cultural place inherently dealing with translations and reinventions of objects that were borrowed from Western science and technology, either as ideas or as direct import products. The "naturalization" of these objects required not only new regulations and ethical codes, but also new rites and rituals, which eventually were transforming the idea of peoples' place in the world. The culture, as I will argue, utilized central social mechanisms so that these life-less bodies could become objects one could give a new name to, speak about, and make part of a rite of passage.[4] If this were somehow not possible, physicians would sink into an endless melancholia about the impossibilities of science in Turkey, or the limits of culture and religion. The efforts of *benimseme* would invent a new identity for these object relations to make them local, familiar, ownable, and legitimately deployable with peace of mind for medical purposes. The local reinvention of these second- or Other-half object relations was as significant as the invention and deployment of these objects for scientific research in the West, as well as their "biotechnical embrace."[5] Only with the new local identity could they be made familiar as noble, legitimate, or useful things and incorporated into social life.

The processes that lead to the invention of this second set of object relations with technological objects profoundly affect the biomedical universe in which people learn to make technology their own. Patients internalize or reject this set of object relations while they try to make sense of the separate worlds they have been a part of. As they spoke to me of impressions from their own pasts, as well as how they thought transplants operated within a machinery of life, patients referred to objects from their pasts as they related to their present changing human condition. Within the limits of social life, the limits of modernity, as well as the limits of the person, technology was changing people's place in life. It was utilizing their past relations to connect worlds otherwise apart in their "new life."

Because these life-less objects were human bodies transformed into commodities by science and technology, I began to think of them through their epistemic qualities. Thus I have staged the ethnography in an epistemic universe in which the "common sense" (*akl-ı selim*) shows the limits of practices, beliefs, and people. Like Clifford Geertz's interpretative anthropology rooted in an extensive understanding of the common sense, I, too, extended my interpretation from common sense toward its dialectical expressions especially to understand belief and its relation to the body. Common sense here refers to the *known,* and its dialectics expressed in the *knowable,* the *unknown,* and the *unknowable,* which are extensions of colloquial or professional deployment of the term.[6] These different epistemic conditions can be seen as acting on many registers, including the *unknowable* metaphysics of life and death, the *known* structure of rituals, and the *knowable* worlds depicted in art and literature, as well as in the *unknown* discovered within scientific discourses.[7] *Akl-ı selim* not only indicates how religious or ethnic differences are drawn, such as the allusive linguistic usages "us" (*biz*) versus "the others" (*ötekiler*), but also shows the roots of Turkish religiosity with shamanism only superficially covered over by Islamic forms. *Akl-ı selim* is like a familiar path providing people with a trail to go further in life through meta-structures and concrete cities. Maybe for this reason, *benimseme* is an essential part of how common sense rules within religious belief systems. I began to think of common sense as the sound way through which the technological objects were made local, so that new external worlds would not appear as alien or strange but as meaningful and familiar.[8] The affective *benimseme* of patients and physicians was profound and resembled the settling down of dust upon a "truth explosion" by which, using common sense, *akl-ı selim*, they tried to make the "new life" their own.

THE BOOK

There are two parts to this book. In part 1, I speak of affect—in this context the mark of technology upon the self that is made desirable. I begin with transplant patients' life histories. From these various life histories, I follow their suffering into larger cultural issues: the lack of brain-dead donors, the so-called organ mafia, the shifting lines between legal and illegal practices, and the institutional power struggles between privatized and public organ-sharing systems and services that patients have been caught in. And from there, I look into the colloquial deployment of the word *kadavra*, the center of transplant politics, which transplant patients and physicians directly borrow from anatomy dissection training and autopsies. Its semiology was a topographic device throughout my fieldwork, one that led me not only to other spheres of medicine but also to crucial spheres of collective life where meaning was produced for and by the transplant patient.

In part 2, I expand on how technological objects are made local. I follow the semiotic implications into "spaces of death," from cemetery to dissection room, from mental hospital back to transplant units, where rituals have been invented by physicians to humanize the *kadavra* and endow them with the moral generosity of donors. In these almost classical forms of ritual process,[9] a new social persona is invented for the *kadavra*, while myths and legends are created to make brain-dead donors bearers of exemplary and purificatory action analogous to sacred sacrifice. As I proceed I situate these semantic slippages, myths, and life histories within the history of modernization in Turkey to understand how a new self-knowledge is born upon relations one has with one's country, community, and family, as well as their interrelatedness, and is carried on through the elements of cultural life such as initiation rites or sacrificial rituals. From the dialysis machine to the metaphors echoing in the machinery of modern life such self-knowledge is produced to stabilize the "truth explosion" and to make patients' uncanny experiences meaningful.

In the conclusion, I look into how these separate worlds, which transplant patients and physicians attempt to suture together, can neither be fully internalized nor rejected by the patient. I write, thus, about the changing self-understanding through technological objects, the post-"truth explosion," patients' limits, their "new life," and *benimseme* as an essential mechanism of our relationship with nature.

IN THE FIELD

The field is never a routine tedious site. One encounters many things at once and thinks of them as a part of the whole body of work, until the moment of filtering, thinning, and refining the material. Before I became fully invested in this topic as a research endeavor, I already had a few initial converging interests and motivations. One was to understand organ trafficking and its place in Turkey, related to matters of human rights, inequalities, and social justice. The other was our changing understanding of death related to ethics of brain-death diagnosis, commodification of the dead body, and the changing metaphysics of life. Probably the most motivating work in giving these interests a form was my reading of Fox and Swazey's classic *Spare Parts: Organ Replacement in American Society* (1992), a work that touched upon the profound affective nature of transplants on the subjectivities of recipients. For reasons that I hope this book will reveal as it unfolds, I also found transplants equally profoundly an intriguing field for exploring our self-understanding of human nature.

To begin with, I was introduced to this topic through two different projects. The first was a summer's fieldwork in Turkey as part of Lawrence Cohen's and Nancy Scheper-Hughes's joint project on global organ trafficking. The second consisted of a year's worth of in-depth interviews with an African American organ donor whose life for me as a Turk opened up an exotic world of Christianity with its powerful commitments to loving sacrifice for family and community. With this experience, my interest in the cultural dynamics of object relations was honed. However, the first project, which provided my initial field material and evoked my interest in the semantics of the *kadavra* was a beginning that would define the structure of my fieldwork in years to come. This was how I began relating the "object relations theory" to my interest in issues of human rights, social justice, and political economy.

The work for Organs Watch was motivating in many ways. While Scheper-Hughes tried to track the illegal and coercive trade worldwide, beginning with Israel, South Africa, Philippines, Moldova, and Brazil, Cohen's work in India was more interested in the epistemic mechanisms of thinking through the regulatory, media, market, and biomedical arenas. Cohen, for instance, showed how the publicity of scandal was deployed and manipulated, how a well-intentioned ban on organ sales helped stimulate an organ market, and how senility and Alzheimer's disease upset pious ideologies about the Indian family and its care of the elderly. My own work aimed to expands the discussion to other spaces beyond the transplant clinic or old age home, tracking a further interlocking set of spaces. Like Cohen, I was interested in the media discourses of scandal, but I wanted to place them also in the context of dramatic changes in legal regulations, newly developed technologies such as an extended viability of kidneys, and the ethical conundrum experienced by all transplant physicians whether tagged as fully legal or not. Like Scheper-Hughes, I too believed that organ trafficking was one of the most troubling violations to the living donor bodies, who were trafficked like slaves. The organ trade, for me, was not necessarily "underground" or "marginal" to local practices, but was rather more of a "business" that came about through medicine's transformation as an inherently economic practice. Organ trafficking happened everywhere; Turkey was no more or no less involved in this kind of "business" than any other neighboring country, or the United States. It was one of the hubs of a large route, which Scheper-Hughes had called the "Kula-ring of organs."[10] In regard to the commodification of the body for medical ends, I began thinking of modernity as producing both a new nation and renewed bodies, as if it were a "business of life,"[11] as something that Foucault might have included under biopolitics.[12] This business was political and first inspired by efforts of the Enlightenment and modernization. It became increasingly economic and was transformed by a neoliberal political economy along with shifting moral understandings such as linguistic shifts that make their users uneasy, competitions over regulatory standards, negotiations over allograft imports, and definitions of brain death within the domestic Turkish cultural economy of affect.

My interest in these problematics deepened as Turkish doctors spoke about the lack of *kadavra*—brain-dead donors. Turkish physicians without an exception thought this to be their main problem. They commonly referred to the example of Japan and Iran, where their colleagues, like them, were hesitant toward brain death. While I was in the field, Margaret Lock published *Twice Dead*, which illustrated in detail the problems Japanese physicians faced acknowledging brain death. Lock emphasized a worldview in which the brain-dead donor whose heart was still beating was hard to naturalize, being both medically dead, as he or she had no cognitive functionality, and yet still living since his or her heart was still pumping blood. I saw similar patterns in Turkey, at least regarding the rigid place the body occupied in cultural sensibilities and in the efforts by physicians, by the Ministry of Health, and by the Presidency of Religious Affairs (Diyanet) to transform it in the public sphere. To understand this better, I followed the semiotic slippages between the cadaver and cadaveric (the word *kadavra* used in both cases) and local understanding of life embodied in words such as *jann*, the life-force, and *emanet*, the body on loan from God.[13]

I saw these semiotic slippages as symptoms of the development of metaphors through which new images and then new objects were being invented. Harriet Ritvo reads the whole of English social life through the invention of taxonomies, which, as semiotic slippages reveal, are only projections of the boundaries of social life. In this sense, semiotic slippages represent the efforts to name not just technological objects but their shifting object relations, and for this reason they occupied the same place in my analysis as taxonomy does for Ritvo.[14]

In the field, I followed these *mindful processes* to places and memories. I wanted to understand how meaning was transferred, translated, or lost. I wanted to find the people behind these translations and losses. That was why I looked into how localities shape difference, form culture, map the flow of capital and politics, and invent in time discourses of ethics—trying to follow a tradition Michael M. J. Fischer introduced in his earlier studies on Iran and later within science studies valuing thick ethnography that could eventually add a new interpretative layer to the already existing political discourses as a way of cultural critique.[15] In a way, time and space, history and locality have become the two constant denominators of my fieldwork method through which people lived and changed.

My central interest in this work has been subjectivity and technology. When I began the initial work on this book as a dissertation project at MIT, I was only one of many on the MIT campus with the same interest. For example, Joe Dumit was writing about personhood understood via imaging technologies. He specifically looked into the interpretation of brain images, where the self was believed to reside or, at least, as courtroom lawyers argue that a positron emission technology (PET) scan can show the difference between normal and abnormal brains; likewise many ordinary Americans used images as part of their "objective self-fashioning."[16] Through the imaging technology, peoples' ideas of the self have changed. Similarly the loss of a kidney could not be understood were it not for technology that provides the necessary imagery and understanding for what it did. One could only lose what one owned; moreover ownership was inherently an epistemic category. Transplant technology, similar to imaging technologies, had to provide the patient with the imagery of an organ in order for the patient to be able to speak of the organ and its loss. Imaginaries of the inner body were the link that connected patients' psychic lives to biotechnology it seemed.

In the case of renal failure, patients learned of the "loss" of an organ as they opened their eyes to a new life after suffering from a coma, and without even understanding what this "loss" would mean to them for the rest of their lives, they were confronted with the dialysis machine. Many of them did not even think of the machine as a permanent life-saving device at that first instant, but as a temporary machine that kept them vital after the renal failure and the following coma. When they were told that they would have to live with the machine for the rest of their lives, that the machine was substituting for their failed renal functions, then they were in shock. Sherry Turkle had spoken of our relationship with machines, with computers in particular, deploying the object relations theory in part, arguing that we change with the machines. Maybe *we* invent them, but they *reinvent* our self-understanding and in this way they change us.[17] The loss of a kidney, the dialysis machine, and the transplant have a similar effect on subjectivity. Like the computer, the robot, or the Internet, the dialysis machine was what Turkle called an "evocative object" that brought out the feelings for the self and for life. People changed as their relationship with life changed through these objects. In their evocations, they began confronting the suppressed or unwanted sides of their personalities in their pasts that eventually lead them to a new self-understanding—a new life.

This new life had two "subjects" in my work: first, patients who abruptly felt changed with the machine or the transplant; and second, physicians who, operating upon a body that belonged to a certain past, country, tradition, and religion, felt they had to appropriate the field in which they introduced this particular technology to operate on the body with the least violation. For this reason, they would launch departments, prepare regulations, open tissue banks, speak of ethical codes of conduct, and even build hospitals to make transplants a "normal" practice. The invention of this universe would allow them to naturalize the imported technology and its objects and make them their own. I will call this universe a "biopolis" in this book to make it a tangible site in which I situate the *collective* life of patients and physicians in a common space and within a biopolitical history.

For physicians, who introduced Western technologies into medical practices, surgery and anatomy dissection were evocative experiences that brought up many social issues, especially those of the marginal, the abandoned, and the loss of communitas. Such surgery and dissection spoke of violence marked upon the physical body, on family relations, and on the inequalities built into the welfare state. The biopolis was the naturalization of the Other through Western technology and someone else's body in the form of an inert self. Nevertheless, this kind of naturalization entailed large and complex problems. While I was trying to make sense of the affect of technology and of patients' transformations in the biopolis, I was deeply influenced by João Biehl's work in Brazil, where he spoke of exclusion and inclusion as "valid" biopolitical categories upon which the politics of life was being construed in a postmodern world.[18] His work with HIV/AIDS patients in Brazil and his study of Catarina, a sufferer of ataxia who was abandoned by her family, were to me powerful examples of people who carried these marks like the transplant patients I had known. From Biehl, I learned to look into the distant corners of social life and beyond the categories "patient," "human," "person," "the insane," and "the cadaver" that were construed upon a certain sense of normalcy. What were the delicacies of culture that naturalized violence, I asked myself. Was Turkey similar to Brazil in regard to postcolonial experiences and abandonment amid inequalities? Was the Turkish case a syndrome of a developing nation? Was comparative or multi-sited ethnography necessary to understand the human condition as it appeared in Biehl's Catarina, or in my Turkish cases of Zehra, Mehmed, or Oğuz in another part of the world? I had seen many parallels: the romantic ways people felt attached to or cut off from life, the physicians who had faith in social justice despite feeling unable to achieve it, the ways Western multinationals had taken over the pharmacologization and medicalization of life, and the ways families could easily abandon loved ones as a survival technique. Biehl's work, in many ways, was an inspiration that allowed me to look into the dark corners of social life where things were left to "another course of life," a domain unwanted, undesirable, or not quite so well fitting to the larger events that changed the material means of single individuals.

Turkey is known for being many things at once. It is a duality of East and West, largely Muslim but with a long Byzantine history of Christianity and a Jewish minority dating back to 1453 and in smaller numbers even earlier. It is a modern nation, but it used to be a powerful empire. It is a democracy, but it has a long tradition of military intervention to protect the secular republicanism established by Atatürk. It is in Europe but also in the Middle East. It is capitalist but with large state holdings. It is neither free of the Western political pressures, like any Middle Eastern country, nor slave to them. It is neither the first world nor a developing nation. It was neither a colony nor a colonizer in the traditional sense of the term, although it was a conqueror of lands from the Balkans and North Africa to the Arabian Peninsula. Turkey is a rich layering of historical horizons piled up, intersecting, dense, and alive. Turkey's pasts encourage one to follow the trails of stories, tales, and legends. New words and new definitions of death would have a hard time finding themselves a suitable place to plant seeds because of its tough soil. People experience life through many invisible elements such as jinn, ghosts, coffee fortunes, and other techniques of the self in their everyday lives, and extend this to other experiences, even to those within realms of reason such as medicine. They understood transplants also through these objects.

Patients I have talked to did not want to survive renal failure no matter the cost. In most cases their main desire was liberation from the dialysis machine, not immortality or a body altered by transplantation that suddenly could not be recognized and trusted as completely their own. From them I learned that organ transplants alter our sense of physical and psychological being like no other technology, literally importing life from one person into the body of another. The recipient's body incorporates the transplanted organ and incorporates along with it all that it embodies and signifies: the life history of the donor, the complicated relationship of the donor with the recipient, the metaphorical and cultural significance of the organ itself and its relationship with the *unknowable,* the high-tech devices that capture the organ and sustain the patient's bodily functions, and the varieties of transplantation policy and politics.

With these things emerges a new consciousness living in, with, and through the body. This experience for transplant recipients is a step beyond the physicians' and researchers' self-referential practice of their vocation in the biopolis, to which I will return below, where metaphors lead to invention of objects and these evoke yet again a new relationship with the world. It more closely resembles fearful paranoia—as well as fragmented, split, schizophrenic conditions—since the object is literally incorporated as a part of the self. It is inevitable, it forces one into transformation. Consequently it is not only psychotic but also transforming. As new distant lives embedded in the invention of the technological object are made part of one's body, the mind opens to worlds that are invisible, suppressed, and unwanted. It bestows a heightened attention to the truth or falsity of the imaginary one inhabits. Some people who experience this change in consciousness feel as if they have entered an altered state designed by some other who has taken over the divine *unknowable* realm.

The experience of a momentous confrontation with an artificial and hence *knowable* world within—replacing the magical and mystical divine—leads to a shift in comprehension. This experience begins with the visualization of the inside of the body, the ability to know the *unknown,* and then goes further deep into the darkness of the soul and finds something familiar and manmade there.

In patients' stories I saw a glimpse of a future when we begin imagining the insides of our bodies with the truth invested in biological knowledge. That, I thought, would be how we begin living a skinless life with a body as an exposed phantasmagoria, an image that reveals a kind of truth other than the elevated sacred knowledge. What is hidden deep inside—impenetrable and solitary, magical and personal—would then become ordinary, visible, and vulnerable, going beyond and beneath the hegemony of an expansive world.

The complex psyche of the person who has received a transplant depends first on the incorporation of the machinic prosthesis of dialysis and then, after the transplant, the internalization and literal incorporation of another's tissue. From patients' experiences it seems as if this altered mental condition and sense of dependence raise consciousness into an undesirable awareness of the artificiality of the world. The affect, which follows from that, seems to stem not from the loss of bodily integrity, but from the loss of *sovereignty*.

Since emotional affect was central to the narratives of transplant patients, that is where I begin, with *benimseme* to understand the "new life." From there I explore Turkish history, poetics, medicine, and politics, then the life of *life-less* objects, and finally the invention of a "second-half" or a "second social persona" for these so that they might reincarnate into a vehicle with healing powers and thus perhaps help transplants become an acceptable practice. In all, step by step, I hope to share the inner workings of cultural processes that give people a new feeling for life and its truth as they find themselves in a biopolis.

PART ONE

THE DESIRABLE

HALF A HUMAN

Oğuz had been having odd sensations since he had been diagnosed with renal failure and began dialysis. These sensations were such that he began to feel as though the dialysis machine took him over, turning him into a robot. After having a transplant, these feelings were replaced with another kind of feeling for his body. As these changes began, he also entered a new realm where he no longer understood himself. All that he could recognize was that he was half: not completely a machine but not completely human either.

Oğuz's health problems started sometime in 1996. He was living with his family in a *gecekondu mahallesi* (slum) of Istanbul where he had joined a gang and had territorial fights with boys from other gangs. One day as he was wandering alone in another neighborhood, he was attacked by twelve or thirteen men and badly beaten for no obvious reason. Covered in blood and with a stabbing pain in his chest, he made his way home. Shortly the pain became so unbearable that he had to go to a small hospital nearby to have it treated. In this privately owned hospital, physicians could not understand the link between the injuries from the fight and the chest pain; they suspected that he was suffering from a lung problem. Since they were unable to make a diagnosis for a couple of weeks, they decided to send him to a big university hospital to be cared for. By then, he had already begun feeling much worse, and then, one day, he collapsed due to internal bleeding. After undergoing a month of tests at the medical school hospital, he was diagnosed with a rare lung illness. In the meantime, however, Oğuz's kidneys had begun failing, and so he began dialysis.

Oğuz did not like the university hospital's dialysis unit. It was not a friendly place; it was a research center and he believed the patients were treated like experimental animals. At least ten different doctors would come by to examine him, each with teams of assistant fellows. They would look at him, touch him, and talk about him as if he were some alien being; they would look into his files and take blood samples, and all of these things made him feel uncomfortable but he had to accept them. Apart from the overwhelming feeling of becoming a research object in the hands of junior physicians, he found dialysis itself a very uncomfortable experience, unpleasant to the point of dehumanization. "*Öldüm öldüm dirildim. Normal insanlıktan çıkmış oldum,*" he said using an expression that literally translates into "I died, I died, and then was resurrected. I exit being a human." His experience was the unbearable *mahrumiyet*—abstinence—from his social life, which he had in common with all other dialysis patients, and with patients in general. His routines enhanced this abstinence.

After dialysis Oğuz would take the public shuttle home and usually throw up at least twice on the way. He could hardly stand when he finally arrived home. The treatment was making his days unbearable, so he decided to go to a dialysis center recommended by his nephrologists. Even though he still felt like he was half-robot, he could at least have meaningful conversations with the staff at the dialysis center. The doctors there were friendly and reassuring. When they talked to him, they did not expect anything in return. He would have tea with the owners—a retired high school teacher and his wife—and they would talk about everyday life or discuss matters that he could not share openly with his own family. In time, the dialysis center became a new home to Oğuz, one where he was welcomed like a son. He no longer threw up after treatment, and instead went home tired but relaxed.

Though treatment at this private center was much more pleasant, being on dialysis nevertheless remained an uncanny experience.[1] It changed the way Oğuz felt about his body and his place in life. If he missed a treatment he would go into a coma; if he were older he could die. He had to be regular and punctual with the three-hour appointments four times a week. When Oğuz realized the importance of the rigid schedule, the restricted life, and his dependency on the machine just to stay alive, he invented his "half-robot, half-human" identity for himself, a joke about his new condition. Attached to the machine, he was like a robot that had to be recharged. The fistula, the plastic tube inserted into an artificial opening in his blood vessel, enhanced his feeling for his machinization—he had to leave the hospital with this small plastic apparatus on his arm, which was like an opening to the outside world. This connection between him and the dialysis machine was open, *açık*, when he was unplugged. He felt open and unguarded.

Through interventions such as this, slowly dialysis taught him what suffering meant. "*Bilmek değil, yaşamak önemli,*" he told me in describing his common sense in another expression, one meaning "What counts is not knowing but lived experience." He would never before have thought that a human could become a robot, an electronic thing. He began to gauge the treatment of his own body in terms of how electronic things should be tended to and cared for. What would happen to a robot, for instance, if one put it in water? It would fall apart, letting off steam and electrical sparks from its exposed wires. And now that he was a robot himself he actually experienced this firsthand. On a beautiful summer day in Istanbul he went swimming after a dialysis treatment. A few days later, wounds like large burns appeared on his back. On a human body wounds like these could be caused not by water but by contact with an electrical current. This strange injury confirmed for him that he was a robot, just like Arnold Schwarzenegger in *The Terminator*—less a person, who would be safe in water, and more a machine, which should not be exposed to it.

There were other physical changes. Like many other dialysis patients, Oğuz had become a hemophiliac. Cuts would take a very long time to heal and wounds would bleed a lot because the blood had been diluted by the dialysis fluid. The dilution even changed the skin's immunity and resistance to cuts. He feared that the connection to the dialysis machine had compromised not only his bodily integrity but also his defense mechanisms, his body's resilience.

Another change was the feeling of an echoing emptiness inside him after dialysis. He felt empty, or rather, emptied out. He was not allowed to drink more than three liters of water between sessions. But he would often drink up to four or five liters, causing his body to swell up. Once the excess water was cycled out of his body by the dialysis, he felt empty. The emptiness inside him—maybe the melancholic feeling of a void—came to be filled by drinking together with his friends, which made him feel that he was just like any other healthy and normal man of his age. He continued the habit even though his doctors and treatment protocol strictly forbade him from doing so.[2] In a secret room behind the local *bakkal*, they drank until the morning hours, causing a greater damage to his body than ever before. He was taking in much more fluid that he was allowed, exceeding his body's limits and causing his health to deteriorate further.

Doctors might have realized and understood his self-destructive behavior, but they never confronted him about it. The nephrologists who cared for Oğuz at the hospital had asked his parents to consider organ donation. His father did the tissue typing and other relevant blood tests and turned out to be a positive match. The nephrologists suggested that Oğuz should receive his father's kidney, but Oğuz did not want it. He was not so sure how a transplant—from his father or anyone else—would improve his life. And had he *known* how it was going to change his life, he would never have accepted it. He would prefer the abstinence at the dialysis machine to the odd psychological transformations that followed the transplant. But he could no longer resist his parents' and the doctors' pressures, and in time he agreed to have the transplant.

The transplant made his relationship with his father worse. As a son who had never been close to his father, he could not bear the transformations. It was as if with the transplanted kidney he had taken in the distance between him and his father. Many feelings about his body emerged with "the kidney," feelings he disliked just as he disliked his relationship with his father. He wished the doctors had told him what it would be like to live with his body like this. But it was not until after the operation, with his father's kidney inside him, that Oğuz was pulled aside by his doctor and told he was not allowed to get married or even have intercourse. The doctor told Oğuz that the new kidney would not last more than nine years, even with the best care.[3] Oğuz would have to be much more attentive to his diet and his lifestyle, because if this kidney failed he would have to live on dialysis for the rest of his life. But on dialysis, he believed, he had had a better life: he could socialize and drink with his friends and then go to dialysis to be cleansed. In a way the machine made it much easier to go on with his social life, compared to the frail transplanted kidney, which demanded constant care. "The kidney" was not his body, nor could it ever become a part of it. It was not a permanent solution. But the dialysis machine was. Knowing these facts, Oğuz began abusing his transplanted body. In time his body would reject his father's kidney anyway, and he could go back to the machine. Why not go back now? Why spend nine years in abstinence?

Oğuz was extremely upset by the new restrictions to his body. Despite much disapproval among his friends, he decided to marry his girlfriend. When he announced that they were engaged, many of his fellow patients became angry with him, telling him it was not his right to destroy the life of a young girl by risking having a baby with her or preventing her from having one. "What if your children suffered from the same disease?" they asked him. "What if you died?" . . . What if he died? What if he died? This was something he did not want to think about any longer; death occupied his mind all the time, taking over his thoughts, possessing him. So one day he decided to take things into his own hands:

So I got something from the pharmacist over the counter. I came home, had a little argument with my parents, and then went to my room. I smoked two cigarettes. I swallowed all the medication. I waited . . . In the meantime one of my parents came in and we had another short argument. . . . I felt my head spinning, so I left home only with my pants on, no shirt, no shoes. I went to the school. In the meantime my mom [having seen Oğuz run out] called all my friends, sent them to look for me. It took them one and a half hours to find me. I had my mobile phone but I didn't answer. If they had been an hour later than they were, we—both the kidney and I (böbrek de ben de)—would have been gone.

Then I started therapy. There [the therapist] asked me odd questions I did not answer. He asked me if I was sexually abused when I was a child. I say no! I say maybe he was abused, not me! I get so upset with his attitude. It is strange . . . when I went there for the first time, I saw six or seven patients with dark circles under their eyes staring into empty space. They looked vacant. Then one asked if I came to see the same doctor. I said yes. Then they said, "Oh welcome, so you are one of us."

Three days later I asked the doctor what medication he gave to his patients that they all looked empty or so dull. I asked him why they were all staying in the same room. He said I was wrong in my assumptions and then he asked the same question about my childhood and sexual abuse. I never went back again. I was there as a normal person; in a week I would become insane like the others. They do strange things, their body language is odd, but in time you start acting like them.

He did not remember exactly why he had wanted to commit suicide. But he was trapped in a life he could not escape; he could not eat or drink or go out and watch a soccer match. Each time he did, his failing kidney forced him into dialysis for a few days. His social life, like his body, had been halved. With the new kidney, he neither lived in a state of biological normalcy as a healthy person nor enjoyed a social normalcy. Even a close friend with whom he had argued one day had yelled at him, "Do not make me angry or I'll punch you, and then you are done with . . . you are just half-a-something anyway! [*yarım kalmış bir şeysin zaten!*]" Oğuz had never forgotten these words; they were carved into his mind like an epitaph. They would constitute his life from then on, confirming his place in the world as truly having become half-a-something. How he felt about his own impairment was one thing, but the fact that others thought he was "half" because he was not physically strong enough to be their equals and to hang out with them was another.

Oğuz was no longer himself; his father's kidney had changed him. He began projecting his negative feelings for his father onto his own body. He used to love the smell of soap—he washed his hands all the time and used up to four or five soap bars a week, playing with it and enjoying its aroma. After the transplant he no longer washed his hands. "For example, I have not washed my hands for two days," he told me one day. "Since the transplantation I cannot wash my hands any longer. If only I knew why. . . . All these habits changed. If I knew why, maybe I could start playing with the soap again." A few months after the transplant, he cut off his distinctive goatee. He was well known for it among his family and friends, and he had been the first to introduce this style to his neighborhood. He had seven different styles for his beard, one for every day of the week. Now he no longer cared about his looks: he didn't iron his trousers or even look in the mirror.

According to his physician, Oğuz suffered from chronic organ rejection, a condition that forces the patient to undergo dialysis every so often even after receiving a transplant in order to keep the new kidney functioning on its own. Oğuz was trying to get rid of the kidney he had been given against his will. His father had taken over his body through the kidney; Oğuz realized he was losing control over himself entirely. He resisted becoming like his father. He lived with his kidney in an absurd symbiotic relationship he could never have *known* or imagined in advance. He could no longer identify with his body, accept it, or like it because of what it had become. The kidney could only be a separate thing attached to him, like his cold and distant father was merely attached to Oğuz's family life. But things had changed and he was grabbed from within; he had lost himself within. Oğuz wanted to be a robot, like the Terminator, even if this meant he would no longer be fully human. It was better than "the becoming" through "the kidney." In the end he had to choose: either to live as half-a-something (*yarım bir şey*) through the dialysis machine, or to die.

FROM THE EARTH, THROUGH THE QUAKE

Hatice suffered renal failure ten days after she gave birth. The overlapping loss and gain, her kidneys and the baby, made her life very difficult in the beginning as she was ill in the hospital and could not care for her baby. But in time, she embraced these things—the failed organ and the new baby—thinking that they were her *nasib* (fate), that they were God's doing.

Her life had been an unfolding surprise in a way. In 1998 Hatice married a sailor who worked for an international shipping company. They had met in İzmit, an industrial town one hour to the east of Istanbul. İzmit's barren concrete landscape is standard third-world imagery—smoke from oil refineries, houses only half-built and leaning into each other to stay upright, many shades of gray looming over laboring workers, and children playing soccer as if they could bring life back to the dying earth beneath the thick concrete of modern life.

It was here that Hatice first met her husband, in a small teahouse facing the sea. Her first impressions were not very positive, so she rejected him like any decent girl would do with an aloof but flirtatious charm. Despite this *naz* (reservation) she expressed, he had sent his mother to meet her parents, an introduction that produced an engagement and then marriage. In time, however, she realized that her first observations were misleading; the man she had married was a wonderful and kind person. Because his work kept him traveling around the world, they could only see each other every forty days or so, when his ship anchored on the Aegean coast in İzmir. She would go there to spend a night on board the ship with him. He would then sail again, usually to America, to New York or Charlestown. Although he was far away for most of the time and she missed him, they had a wonderful life whenever he got time off to spend a whole month together,.

Hatice's husband was just back from another long trip to stay with her for a month early in August 1999. They had made plans to spend time with their families and then go on a vacation. But on August 17, two weeks after her husband's arrival from America, misfortune came about: they were awakened in the middle of the night by thundering noises rising up from the depths of the earth and into their bedroom. At the sound Hatice jumped out of her bed, grabbed her clothes and handbag, and managed to escape down the stairs, holding her husband's hand. As they were rushing out, throughout the whole city the earth was shaking, and then seconds later its surface ripped apart like a sheet of paper. The frail squatter homes that hundreds of thousands of İzmit's people had built upon its concrete landscape slid into the depths of the earth. Hatice and her husband were saved. However, their lives, like those of so many others who lived close to the epicenter, would no longer be the same after this momentous shock.

Outside their building many people waited, half-naked and fearful, afraid to go back to their apartments even after the shaking stopped. They huddled together. As the sun rose and the aftershocks seemed to subside, they could see a new era beginning in their street, their neighborhood, their city. It was a new era for the whole country, and it had announced itself on that day by taking many lives, most of them poor, and by tearing the concrete open and leaving the souls of the dead trapped under the wreckage instead of letting them ascend into the fresh summer air.

The appropriate funerary rites of passage have never been completed for these lost masses. Instead those dead bodies were absorbed into the moment to be remembered as the *deprem* (the earthquake), just as they diffused into the bodies of those who survived, penetrated into the water people drank, and decayed into the earth people walked on, instead of entering the heavens. They were buried everywhere in the thin layer between God's *unknowable* heaven and the earth's dark bosom. For some it was reminiscent of the Day of Judgment. For others, it was as if the earth had released a deep-seated energy and in exchange swallowed fresh cool bodies.

Relief efforts began immediately, though the politicians argued over the announcement of the disaster, whose aid to accept, and what private hospitals to open to the public. As the day proceeded, the scale of this massive turning point for the country become clearer. The death toll was first announced as a few hundred, but in a matter of hours it was raised to a few thousand, and in the days to come to tens of thousands, as if a veil had been lifted while the government tried to hold back the real numbers.

In the midst of this mess Hatice and her husband began living in Kızılay (Red Crescent) tents together with many of the others who were not allowed to enter their damaged homes. Around ten days after the quake, she thought she might be pregnant; she took a test and it came out positive. Despite the horrors of life in the tents, the smell of corpses, and the aftershocks, she and her husband were happy. But unpredicted threats followed one after the other. A few nights after they learned she was pregnant, an LPG tank at the nearby refinery in Petkim caught fire and almost exploded. Not able to stay so close to the refineries, they rushed to the mountains to seek shelter with everyone else. They were allowed to come back to the ruins the next day after the fire had been brought under control. The dusty roads were packed with trucks full of soldiers, people searching for their lost families, rescue workers trying to help, and the media trying to get a glimpse of the drama.

People get used to things. Like any other disaster that reduces individuals to tiny specks of dust in a vast universe of forgotten things, this one eventually slowed its pace. In time, people internalized their suffering, made it part of their lives.

Hatice and her husband went back to their home only to move to a safer place close to Hatice's mother. From her family, two of her cousins were killed in the quake but the rest were in good health. As things returned to normal, she realized this was their *nasib*—their share of destiny—they could not have prevented or changed it. Most importantly, observing the suffering of so many people, she realized that the earthquake was not an individual punishment but a collective experience. She went back to normalcy together with everyone else, talking about it, remembering it, and slowly transforming its memory into one of those events one remembered occasionally.

The months of her pregnancy were the months of the nation's recovery from the shock of the earthquake. The overwhelming experience may have made her hospital visits a challenge. Preparing for birthing, she went to a gynecologist who was merely interested in her pregnancy and not her general health. Hatice did not think of telling a gynecologist about her kidney stones. The birthing turned out to be very difficult and resulted in a cesarean section. Afterward she fell ill—she could not even drink the *lohusa şerbeti* (a traditional sweet, spiced iced tea that is believed to help women produce breast milk)—and began throwing up constantly as her legs swelled. Ten days later, she was in a coma.

She opened her eyes to find her body connected to a dialysis machine. At first she did not even understand why. She thought the machine was for life support. Then she was told that her kidneys had failed, that she had to be on dialysis for the rest of her life. Because she was so ill, they had taken away her daughter and given her to her mother for care. In the six months that followed this beginning, she would think and rethink about what was happening to her.

As she began the routine of the machine with other dialysis patients her life had become a challenge: she was alone in this, no one else from her neighborhood went to dialysis with her and it took so much of her time and energy that she could no longer take care of her baby. She no longer lived a normal life. "This is *nasib*," she said. "One should not get upset about things. Having hope that things will get better is the best way to deal with it. See, now I am having a transplant, and I will be normal again. I will be the only one who goes though such a thing in my family."

Living in a large family made difficulties less apparent and her burden lighter. Hatice had nine siblings, of which she was the fourth. During those months of meditation on her new physical constitution, it did not occur to her to consider having a kidney transplant. The waiting list for organ sharing was very long. One of her friends from dialysis had been on it for four years. Hatice thought she could look into other ways of recovery such as taking herbal supplements for comfort and relief. There was a prominent herbalist *hoca* (spoken as *hodja*, healer) in Eskişehir. She visited him with her husband. The herbs she got were tasteless and stank; they did not give her the relief she had hoped for. But on seeing what Hatice was going through merely to have a normal life, her mother had compassion for her. She took the tissue typing and blood tests to see if she could donate a kidney to Hatice. So began the story of her transplant. All of Hatice's sisters took the tests too, and two were a match. Hatice was glad. This was *nasib*, she thought. Who would have thought her life could change like this? She owed her sister her life. Her sister was unmarried. With one kidney missing her sister would not be allowed to have more than one child. Hatice was so grateful for her sister's generosity that she promised to pay her dowry or to help her in any way she could.

"It is a relief to be liberated from the machine. I will be normal again. It is not nice to live on a machine. The dialysis machine has all this wiring that goes in and out, the dirty blood goes out of you and the clean blood comes in. It is like a washing machine," she said smiling. Her fistula had closed right after she had the transplant. She was a little sad about it. The little buzzing apparatus had become a part of her, and she took care of it diligently to keep it clean and open. She showed it to her friends, who were puzzled by the tiny shock they would feel when they touched it. With her sister's kidney working properly in her body, her wish had come true.

Now that she was recovering from a life of abstinence, Hatice had one more thing to finish: a vow she had to fulfill now that she was liberated from the machine. God had answered her prayers, but she was already beginning to feel depressed in the hospital because she was unable to complete her obligation and sacrifice an animal in thanks. To free her mind of this burden she asked her parents to do it for her. They sacrificed a lamb, which they then donated to charity (because one is not allowed to consume the meat of animals sacrificed for the fulfillment of a personal petition). With the sacrifice completed, Hatice relaxed. Everything was set. God had answered her prayers, she had kept her promise, and the order of things had been reestablished. She would take care of her daughter, her sister's kidney, and her sister, which were all hers now to look after, they were her *nasib*.

Nasib, in the end, was about having one's share in a collective experience: it forced one to accept the unexpected given. It required adjustment of life. Besides, one gave away something in exchange for something else. And if this exchange concerned *jann* (life-force), like in Hatice's case, it meant she would have to mobilize rites that mediated between worlds, the next one from which the *nasib* came and this one, in which it was to be transformed into a normalcy in everyday life. Hatice's kidney was an object like this.

As she shared the terrors of the earthquake with her family and neighbors, she must have taken a piece of that drama within and lost her kidney. This drama would mark the beginning of her new relationship with the *unknowable* divine, who had taken away her own kidney but gave her a baby and a new kidney.

AGAINST THE TIDE

When Fidan was diagnosed with kidney failure, she believed it was the end of her life as she knew it. She lived in Balıkesir, a city close to İzmir, where she had a vivid life filled with social gatherings, friendships, and many acquaintances. But the renal failure took away all that she was so proud to be a part of. After her diagnosis, she retreated into a solitary existence for two years. She isolated herself from her friends, did not accept any guests, visit any friends, talk to people on the street, or greet her own neighbors. She would draw the curtains as soon as she arrived home. She would close in behind curtains and doors. As her health deteriorated, Istanbul awaited her with its specialists and hospitals. She left her hometown like a ghost, not announcing her departure and without a farewell party. She could not say goodbye. Words failed her.

In Istanbul, she spent four more years on dialysis, but these years were not as difficult as the beginning years in her hometown of Balıkesir, where she did not want to or could not share her ill health with her friends, where the lost kidney had to be some sort of a secret. Then in time, Fidan realized she had to get used to this new situation, accept her body, and continue her life as usual.

Despite her desire to lead a normal life, she had become depressed on the dialysis machine and unable to enjoy life. She no longer followed fashion, read recipes, or cooked like she used to. She wanted to study, learn, and do more things with her life. Shortly before the kidney failure, she had taken university entrance exams and gotten into the Open University in Eskişehir. She could get a university degree by taking courses via television from home. This would be her chance to study since she was not allowed to go to the university because of the ban on the headscarf. After the kidney failure, however, she no longer wanted to do it—not because of lack of time but lack of will.

The loss of a kidney came along with isolation and depression, but it also enhanced the richness of her family life. At home, Fidan's family was always by her side. Her husband cooked, her children helped around the house, her own mother opened her home to her family when they spent their first year in Istanbul, and then after she moved to a new apartment with her family, her relatives came over to help her clean. The support she received from her loved ones was overwhelming, yet she still could not accept her new life. The dialysis made her only half-human.

> [The] real illness is being on dialysis. . . . It was a disaster for me. I could hardly accept it. In dialysis I would not talk to anyone. You lose your faith in life, you do not want to buy new clothes, you do not want to go out. You do not take pleasure in anything. This continued for two years. On the first day we fear something (*içimizde korku var*). . . . I could guess about how the machine works. I had read about it. I was thinking of the impact of the machine on my heart. Would it have side effects? It damages the body. . . . I do not like complaining much. I have children and family. . . . I did not know what would happen to them. So your attitude to life changes.

Though the dialysis was a very difficult experience, it was not her first challenge in life: it actually reminded Fidan of the way she struggled with the issue of the headscarf. Fidan grew up in a household with conservative values where women traditionally wore a headscarf.[4] Symbols of religion, such as the headscarf, the veil, and the beard used to be forbidden in public service in Turkey because they were considered to be signs of political resistance to the secular principle of the republic and the modernist values of progressive and open nationhood. However, the ban on headscarves had a paradoxical effect; though intended to emancipate women and to ensure the right to education, the ban prevented women like Fidan from participating in public education.

Fidan's life was an imprint of these social problems. They constituted her everyday experience. She believed that the ban was a violation of her personal expression; the state presumed that everyone who covered her head was a criminal. It was as if a woman wore the headscarf to conceal the anti-authoritarian and rebellious political ideas that were in her mind; it was as if by uncovering (*başını açmak*) she would automatically become innocent. Would a person's ideas change when she took off the headscarf? No. But the state had made the public believe that would be the case. Fidan, like many others, felt oppressed by this manmade machinery, the modern state, which she believed wanted to transform her belief system by labeling her headcovering as a countersymbol to progressive modern social life in Turkey. Over the years, she had slowly developed a certain dislike of the state. The rising inequalities among people, the never-ending debates on the right to education, and the headcovering all gradually caused her to feel that the history related in history books telling mythic tales of national heroes was unreliable.

One of Fidan's sisters went to England to pursue her master's degree in psychology because she could not attend school in Turkey while wearing a headscarf. The state's oppressive regime against covering was *haksız*—unjust—for its citizens. It was actually more than unjust, she thought: it was *zulüm*—oppression, persecution, cruelty. Fidan did not like being viewed as a potential criminal or an outcast—who would? Her mind was not devoid of disagreements, but her headscarf did not cover a conspiracy. Yet the state placed her in the categories of criminal and outcast, and people learned to know her through them. Life at dialysis, by analogy, was a similar categorization. She was no longer equal to others. This time, at dialysis, she was literally different. And this time, she felt that oppression had materialized in the form of a dialysis machine and kept her behind others. She depended on this machine to be alive like she depended on the state to be a person, to be able to do things, to study or to work.

She met many in her dialysis unit who, like her, had lost faith in life. They did not have much hope in their future. She did not want to relate to them. All that she wanted was to liberate herself from the machine (*makinadan kurtulmak*) as she worded it using a phrase commonly invoked by dialysis patients. This could not be her new community, her new family, her new life. The thought of it depressed her more than anything else. She had to change something so she decided to list her name in the organ-sharing database in Istanbul for a cadaveric kidney transplant.

Most people were encouraged to get kidneys from their family members or close kin. In her case, she was unable to do so. She had nine siblings, all of whom were married with children. She could not ask any of them for a donation. In fact, none of them had approached her. Instead, they had offered her money—each as much as he or she could afford—so that she could buy herself a kidney in the illegal market. Besides getting a kidney from a brain-dead donor, buying seemed to be her only option.

Yet, life is for people (*hayat insanlar için*), as she worded it. A tragic illustration of this arose suddenly in Fidan's family. Her sister—the psychologist who had faced difficulties with the headscarf—died in a car crash. She was young; her unexpected death was a blow to the whole family. She had told Fidan long ago that if anything happened to her and she died suddenly, Fidan could have her kidney. She would not need it in the grave, would she? One's organs rotted in the earth, anyway. Why waste them if they could save someone's life? Did it not say in the Qur'an that saving one life meant saving the life of all beings? Fidan meditated on her body and matters of life and death, suffering in dialysis, and what awaited her when she died. Thinking about taking her sister's kidney at a time of mourning was hard. But she did think about it eventually; she remembered that it was her sister's legacy, that she had donated her kidneys to Fidan. Unfortunately, the body was too damaged and there had been no brain-death diagnosis.[5] It would have been impossible to use her sister's kidney, even if Fidan had tried to act on it right away in the midst of her grief.

Fidan's suffering was unbearable. She started seriously considering buying a kidney. There was much talk in the dialysis unit about where to find them, and she could not help but listen to the stories: "I thought of going abroad. Russia or Iraq. . . . We heard it is not so hygienic there. You learn it from patients. I talked to a patient who has been abroad. There are companies who do this, some you cannot trust. . . . You hear people go there, some die on the [operating] table. I think their corpses must be brought back. The companies must be doing that. . . . It is a problem."[6] Fidan could never really make the effort to find out more about it though. It was less an issue of illegality and more of her mistrust in the management of the companies and the treatment of dead bodies in foreign lands. What if she died abroad? What would happen to her body there?

Organ selling did not bother her as far as morality was concerned. The state was corrupt and was run by people who allowed only the privileged to profit. Simple people like herself would always suffer under its oppressive regulations. Organ trafficking and the headscarf issue were both examples of this. How could she trust the state? Its agenda was muddled by its alienation from simple people. She had to learn Arabic to read the Qur'an, and with her knowledge of Arabic script she could also read Ottoman. She realized how people's memories had been erased from one day to the next with the reformation of the alphabet in 1926. One could not even read cookbooks from the past. One day Turks were reading and writing in the Orient in Arabic letters and the next day their minds were in the Occident with the Latin alphabet. "Our links with history were cut off with it [the Arabic alphabet]: it is like being on dialysis. One day you live normal, the next day you are cut off from life."[7]

Fidan could not but live dialysis life through the politics of the modern state. Like life had abandoned her, Turkey had abandoned its heritage, its memory, its language, and its identity, becoming another country altogether. The state pretended to maintain normalcy by erasing memory, writing a new history, and banning free thought. And in this agenda, Fidan was not a part of the country's body, but of its malady.

Despite her disregard for the state's laws, she did not want to get involved in organ trafficking. Besides, she was worried about the hygiene conditions abroad. She kept on waiting. And then one day, quite unexpectedly, she received a phone call from the hospital. There was a kidney from a nine-year-old boy who was diagnosed with brain-death after a car crash and the medical evaluations matched her profile—she could have the kidney. The operation was successful and since then she has felt reborn. As she found the strength to live, her future appeared and she began her "reborn" life back in her own privacy, her *mahrem*.[8]

TRAVELING TO THE WEST AND THE EAST

In 1982, when he was twenty-seven years old, Sedat married his high school sweetheart, Aysel, in a small family ceremony. As they were just beginning to plan their lives, two months after their wedding, he was hospitalized because of fever and pain. At the hospital he was told that his kidneys were failing, that he had to begin dialysis treatment. This was a time when transplants from living-related donors were a new practice for Turkish transplant surgeons. For patients who wanted to have a transplant instead of waiting for long years for a brain-dead donor those were even more experimental years.

Both Sedat and Aysel had finished high school in 1974, a year of political upheavals; many students and workers in left- and right-wing groups clashed with the police and with each other in the university every day. Sedat fled the town to escape the everyday violence and began his mandatory military service while Aysel continued studying. By the time he came back from the military she had already finished university and had been assigned to teach in Van in eastern Turkey. They got married right away so that they could apply to have her mandatory service as a teacher switched to Istanbul, but it took them a year to complete the paperwork. In the meantime Sedat had moved to Istanbul and found work as a sailor. Working hard, he quickly had earned a promotion to a position as the private assistant to the ship's wealthy owner. In time, the owner would become like family. When Aysel came back from Van to start teaching in Istanbul, their relationships had become so close that Sedat's boss wanted to pay for the post-wedding party that they had planned on throwing in Istanbul. Unfortunate events, however, followed this lovely beginning: two months after Aysel's arrival in Istanbul, Sedat's kidney ailments began. He had caught cold from the strong Bosporus winds while working in the harbor—he had felt the cold crawling up his back every so often. At first he was diagnosed with nephritis—infection of the kidney.

The infection was treated, but Sedat had to begin dialysis as well. His boss had learned of Sedat's deteriorating health and showed much kindness and generosity, assuring Sedat that he would not lose his job and that the company would take care of his medical expenses if insurance did not cover them. Sedat felt very fortunate.

At home, living at his parent's place with Aysel, and having just married, Sedat lived a life filled with the routines and restrictions of a large family. Sedat's siblings and his mother wanted to donate a kidney to him right away, but the test results did not indicate a match, and he was unable to receive a kidney from any of his close kin. His only chance seemed to be a cadaveric transplant. But back in the mid-1980s cadaveric donations were very rare in Turkey. Organ transplantation was still in its initial stages and was not widely practiced. In 1987, Prime Minister Turgut Özal's newly re-elected government had drafted legislation permitting Turks to go abroad to seek organ transplants and subsidizing their living and medical expenses. This was supposed to be extended to everyone regardless of level of income or connections, but somehow not everyone was able to get the paperwork processed.

After months of making inquiries and processing the paperwork, Sedat managed to get his name listed for the insurance allowance abroad. England was then a common destination for Turks in need of specialized health-care services. His doctors in Istanbul supported the idea, and in no time he and his wife were on their way to London. The Turkish state had granted them a monthly stipend of over £2,000, which was a small fortune back then in part because they stayed with relatives in the suburbs of London and did not have to spend money on rent. The first six months of their stay in London were nice. Sedat got listed on an organ-sharing list, and while waiting for the matching kidney to save his life he and his wife did some sightseeing and even some shopping.

After months of waiting, however, there was no sign of a cadaveric kidney. Sedat was persistent, and seeing this, his doctor at the London clinic approached him with a surprising question: would his wife consider donating a kidney to him if she were a match? Sedat had not come all the way to England to receive his own wife's kidney—he wanted a cadaveric organ. But the doctor tried to persuade him: there were two other Turkish couples who had arrived in London at the same time as Sedat and Aysel; they could all have the operation together. To Sedat, this suggestion was disturbing. What if they took his wife's organ and transplanted it into someone else? What if he were given a less worthy organ instead? If such a thing did happen, no one [of the Turkish community at the same hospital] would know what was going on because they would all be in the surgery room at the same time.

The English physician left him with no other alternative as time passed. After a while, Sedat agreed. The test results indicated a match, and instead of getting a cadaveric kidney from an English donor, Sedat received his wife's kidney in London—an operation he could as well have had in Turkey. The imposition troubled him a lot, but he felt they did have not much choice left as months passed.

Sedat's initial paranoia about corruption was not ungrounded. His fears materialized soon after his operation. The police discovered that the physicians in that clinic were involved in organ trafficking. They were harvesting organs from illegal Turkish immigrants and transplanting them into patients who traveled there from Israel and elsewhere. The Turkish embassy called in all the Turks from the hospital to inquire about their treatment. The head surgeon was taken into police custody. With this very disturbing news, Sedat's adventure in London ended. They went back to Istanbul as soon as they could with Sedat carrying his wife's kidney inside him.

Aysel's kidney worked well for Sedat for three and a half years. He was in good health except for his emotional life, but for some obscure reason he began neglecting his post-transplant treatment and did not want follow the required medical procedures, which were so vital in a post-transplant life. As he sank into a kind of depression, he was convinced that he had received the wrong kidney from the English doctor, and that his wife's healthy kidney had been transplanted into a wealthy patient—that he had been given a kidney from a stranger. He was confused, aggressive, depressed. As time passed he became a tyrant at home: he yelled at Aysel, humiliated her, never showed kindness. He did not understand the cause of his sudden eruptions. Was this not the woman who had given him her kidney, who had traveled with him all the way to England? Was she not the mother of his child? She had shown him such generosity; she had saved his life yet he could not live with her kidney. In time, the kidney began failing him. And then it failed entirely. In 1992 he began dialysis again because the failed kidney had been removed.

Back in England, Sedat and his wife had saved most of their state allowance. Later on in Istanbul, those savings had become a small fortune, enough to buy two apartments in the suburbs of the city back then. But Sedat still preferred living with his parents, despite his wife's efforts to convince him to move out to a place of their own. In time their London savings were spent, and they were again left with nothing of their own except for a car. Sedat's family life worsened as money grew scarce. With the kidney failure and those long draining dialysis sessions, he had become even more dependent on his family—a condition he could no longer take. He felt he had to begin a new life yet again. He thought what they really needed was their privacy, a family life of their own, so they moved out of his parents' place. Finally, for the first time in his life he and his wife finally could be on their own in their own home.

With the beginning of this renewed family life, Sedat decided to try again in 1995. This time he could go to Russia to have a cadaveric transplant. Times had changed. What used to be Turkey's northern neighbor—the Soviet Union, the home of left-wing inspiration for Turkish intellectuals and the student movements of the 1960s and 1970s—had become an independent state easily accessible to Turkey. Commercial treaties now linked the two countries, especially in construction. A new mobility spawned partnerships in many kinds of business. Immigrants from former Soviet republics started pouring into Turkey; some were investors, some were laborers, and some were prostitutes. In this emerging trade zone, people wanted to make money quickly. Medium-sized companies had seen this as an opportunity for expansion, traders had seen this as a chance to bring products of labor (bodies included) from one country to the other. Small traveling companies emerged in the shadow of this boom and moved people along these routes. Before long, the middle-class medical patient had joined the crowd in search of treatment opportunities. Poverty, mobility, and the lifting of the iron curtain made the mingling of cultures and bodies visible across sections of social life that had been previously invisible; the transnational had opened a new realm for possibilities of a reborn life.

Likewise, Sedat kept hearing stories about transplants in Russia. In Sedat's dialysis unit, one of the doctors knew how to contact a company—the doctors were actually being paid a small fee by the agency for providing its information to dialysis patients. With this physician's recommendation, Sedat met the company owner, who was married to an Azeri woman fluent in Russian. She would accompany the patients on the trip, serve as their translator, settle them in the hospital, and see to it that everything was done properly.

For this trip, however, Sedat could not take his wife. They had spent most of their savings. It would be expensive to live in Moscow for an indefinite period of time. The Turkish state no longer covered such expenses, and Sedat would end up spending the equivalent of U.S.$27,000 (in 1996) for this operation.

Sedat went to Moscow twice for the transplant. During his first visit, the doctors sent him back home to be treated for tuberculosis—an illness he had suffered from as a teenager. In the meantime, the owner of the travel agency was arrested on charges of smuggling patients and illegal immigrants. Despite this slight complication, Sedat was soon back on a plane with the owner's Azeri wife. This time, however, he was the only patient on the plane. As soon as they landed, he was taken to a private hospital in downtown Moscow. There he would meet six other Turkish patients, among them Aziz, who would become his closest friend—a story I tell below. In this hospital, Sedat met people from around the neighboring countries, including Germans but also many people from the young republics that had emerged with the fall of the Soviet Union.

Sedat was not happy in Moscow. The food was not good: he could not find *helâl* meat, so he abstained from meat and switched to a vegetarian diet. Over months of waiting for a transplant, this new diet caused his health to deteriorate. Sometimes he and his friend Aziz would go to eat at McDonald's—the fast-food restaurant chain—since he did not want to eat the hospital food because of cultural differences in diet. In addition to the food problems, he had to get used to living the long summer days, from 4 AM to midnight, an unfamiliar biological cycle. The only time he could rest was during those few hours of darkness at night. But the worst of all was waiting day after day for the matching kidney. All of the transplant patients who were there before him had already received transplants and left. Four times the doctors told him there was a kidney available; each time he would have his hopes up, but then it would turn out to be a mismatch. He was slowly becoming demoralized as a result.

After months of unbearable waiting, at last "a kidney arrived" from Leningrad. On the verge of a complete breakdown, Sedat had the transplant. His friend Aziz was still there for him even though he had had his operation already. Unfortunately, despite the biologically apparent match, Sedat's new kidney did not work. With the new kidney inside, he was back on dialysis again. He did not suffer from an immune rejection, but neither was the kidney functioning properly.

Sedat stayed at the hospital for two more months without any hopes of recovery. And then one day, when he was up on the fifth floor of the hospital building, he thought of committing suicide. What was there left for him? He had lost a lot of weight, most of the Turks he had met in Russia had already left, he had no one to talk to, there was no television, and his wife could not visit him. He was a sickly man, dependent on a machine, living far away from everything he loved. The hospital was like a prison. One day, he climbed up to a large window and looked down. With a little step, he could end his life. But then, suddenly, he remembered his mother, his sisters, and his beloved wife, who had given him her kidney to save his life. What would they do if they learned he had died in a foreign land? They would suffer for the rest of their lives. He could not hurt them like that. He backed away from the window.

Sedat's stay in Russia drew on. His depression had not escaped the attention of his doctor, who approached him with kindness and told him to go back to Turkey. "You will never recover here. . . . If you don't eat any meat or any food, your wounds will not heal," the doctor advised. He was right. There was nothing more they could do to help improve Sedat's health in Moscow. He had to go back to Istanbul to his family, to his wife. By then he had been in Russia for six months already.

He announced his arrival date to his family. His wife and his sister were waiting for him impatiently at the airport to pick him up. When he arrived he almost fainted in their arms. He had to be hospitalized right away, but it was hard to find an open dialysis center on a Sunday. After they found out that the dialysis unit at the Istanbul University Medical School Hospital (Çapa) was open, they had to convince the doctors there to take care of Sedat. The physicians were reluctant to take on a patient who had just arrived with a nonfunctioning transplant from Russia. Sedat had to agree to the physicians' terms: that he was solely responsible for the operation in Moscow, that no doctor from the unit at Çapa had done any harm to him, and that if he suffered another organ rejection there they would not be held responsible for it. And so he was admitted to Dr. Uluğ Eldegez's transplant unit. Two days later, doctors surprised him with the good news. His test results were fine. The kidney was working and healthy and he no longer needed to be on dialysis. Still, Sedat had other ongoing health problems: his lungs were swollen with five kilograms of water and he had tuberculosis. He stayed in Çapa's intensive care unit (ICU) for another four months. After this long medical journey of almost one year, he could finally go back home to his wife and his daughter. His Leningrad kidney has been working fine ever since.

He no longer minded the prospect of going in for dialysis again—he knew that transplant kidneys never lasted a lifetime. But some sort of a miracle had happened to him since his last transplant. He had changed. When he looked back, he could not understand why he had been such a difficult man, a "fascist" as he worded it, while all the while his wife was trying to support him. With the Leningrad kidney, he was himself again.

WITHIN THE EXPERIMENT

Each thought, each day, each life lies here as on a laboratory table. And as if it were a metal from which an unknown substance is by every means to be extracted, it must endure experimentation to the point of exhaustion. No organism, no organization, can escape this process. Employees in their factories, offices in buildings, pieces of furniture in apartments are rearranged, transferred, and shoved about. New ceremonies for christening and marriage are presented in the clubs, as if the clubs were research institutes. Regulations are changed from day to day, but streetcar stops immigrate too. Shops turn into restaurants and a few weeks later into offices. This astonishing experimentation—it is here called *remonte*—effects not only Moscow, it is Russian.

—WALTER BENJAMIN, *Moscow Diary*

Aziz felt the spirit of *remonte* deep inside when he, like Sedat, went to Moscow for a cadaveric transplant at the same hospital. He thought that the hospital was surrounded by cold pompous buildings that were remnants of the Communist regime, and lively markets, which now were in the hands of an emerging mafia. To Aziz, Moscow had huge avenues with a *ruhsuz mimari* (soulless architecture). There were no shop windows. Instead, apartments in big Communist-era housing complexes had been converted into shops but still were unidentifiable as places of commerce. Newly emerging street markets and shopping malls were expanding alongside these strange commercial areas. There was much poverty on the streets: not like the poverty in Turkey, which deprived people from buying books, he thought, but widespread poverty, poverty as a basic human condition.

The hospital was likewise poor yet it had a separate floor for private operations for people like him coming from abroad. The company that brought Turkish patients to Moscow for transplants lodged them in hospitals with such private floors—three different places in the city. It was a legitimate business, even to the extent that after Aziz returned to Turkey he and his "Russian kidney" were featured in a local newspaper. In this quasi-legal environment, it was hard to tell the difference between the apartment and the shop, the mafia and the state, the hotel and the hospital. It was an exciting time to be in Moscow, but a difficult time to be a foreign patient there, in the chilly hospital in the hands of "travel agents" whose work was neither legal nor really illegal.

But before Moscow, Aziz too had been to different places to recover from a deteriorating health condition caused by renal failure. He was thirty-nine years old when his kidney failed. This was in 1992, soon after he got married. He had been undergoing treatments for diabetes by then, and one day he felt miserable and rushed to the hospital with complaints of nausea. At the time, it did not cross his mind that this visit would mark the beginning of a dramatic change in his life: the diagnosis at the ER indicated renal failure.

After this diagnosis, Aziz packed his luggage and left for Florida right away. He had a physician friend there working as a nephrologist and Aziz could stay at his friend's boss's house. He was there four days. They ran tests, including a biopsy, which they hoped would explain his sudden renal failure and show them how damaged his kidneys were so that they could plan Aziz's treatment. The results, however, were not encouraging: the American doctors thought Aziz had a genetic inclination toward kidney failure. Aziz was upset: he was ill and he had to be treated right away. The genetic information would not help him with a treatment. His parents had both passed away. His father had died from diabetes and other related ailments. Forty days after his father's death, his mother suffered a heart attack and died. He had no siblings. He knew that his paternal grandparents had also died suddenly and at a young age, maybe also because of kidney failure. He was depressed about this lack of medical history, of any records of his family's biological past, except his knowledge of the diabetes they all suffered from.

Aziz decided to follow the American doctors' advice to start on peritoneal dialysis, a treatment he could prepare at home or in his office by himself. Feeling much worse than ever before, he decided immediately to go back to Turkey to discuss his condition with his physician friends there. All the flights to Istanbul were sold out when he arrived at the airport. He could not tell the ticket agents about his illness; he knew they would not allow him on board. With the urea in his blood increasing, his body swelling, and his blood pressure increasing he could not wait another twenty-four hours for the next available flight. He had to go back to the hospital. The next morning, after a few phone calls, he decided to fly to Houston and take a Lufthansa flight from there to Istanbul via Frankfurt. He departed from Florida to Houston and arrived there in much pain. The Lufthansa flight was not for another eight hours.

In these everlasting eight hours, Aziz thought he had come to the end of his journey in this world. He could hardly stand, sit, eat, or drink. He believed he would die very soon.

Yet, after eight hours of a phantasmagoric wait, he got on that Lufthansa flight and made it back to Istanbul. He landed at midnight the next day and went directly to the hospital for dialysis. He was back. It was great to have cleansed blood. In time he got on to the peritoneal dialysis at home and at work, following its six-hour cycles and the strict hygiene guidelines, knowing however that he could not go on living that way. In the United States he had been advised to consider a transplant right away as he had been told that the longer he remained on dialysis the weaker his immune system would become.

Having lost all of his family, his only chance for a new kidney was to buy one. But before he planned on a venture of this kind, he decided to talk to some hospital administrators to see how he should proceed. His first visit was to Ankara. He had a meeting with Dr. Mehmet Haberal, who in the space of a couple of minutes listed the requirements for a transplant in his hospital: Aziz should either find a living-related donor and have the operation in Haberal's hospital, or drop his name from Istanbul's organ-sharing waiting list for a cadaveric transplant, and sign up on Haberal's organ-sharing list in Ankara instead. Haberal's requirements were hard to meet. Aziz would have to quit his job in Istanbul and move to Ankara if he decided to have the transplant there. Besides, the meeting with Haberal lasted only a few minutes, far too short to establish a proper patient-doctor bond with such a difficult matter at stake.

After seeing Dr. Haberal, Aziz met with Dr. S. Back then in the mid-1990s Dr. S. had not yet become Turkey's famous "organ mafia" doctor, nor had he yet acquired his reputation as "Robin Hood" among some dialysis patients. Dr. S. had a reasonable pricing scale and told Aziz that he could provide him a kidney from India for U.S.$25,000. Aziz was not thrilled about this plan. In 1995, the Indian organ market was at its peak, but many transplant patients suffered complications in the post-transplant phase due to low hygiene conditions during the operation. Dr. S. calmly told Aziz how he should prepare himself psychologically for an operation like this. His advice had a deep impact on Aziz. He began viewing transplants with a new perspective and could prepare himself to internalize the kidney he eventually would get. Dr. S. had told him all the possible psychological stages he might go through after the operation—how he should embrace them and face the challenges they presented. What Aziz learned during that meeting kept him strong throughout his transplant experience, and without these in mind, he believed, he would not have managed to hold onto life.

Of the few options he had been presented with, Aziz choose to follow the least ethically and medically challenging one he could. One of his friends from work had had a transplant in Moscow, which sounded to Aziz like the most appealing option. If he had to choose between India and Russia, he preferred the "Russian solution." In Russia, he was told, all corpses belonged to the state, a fact that made a large number of transplants possible. Russians, he thought, must have good medical expertise remaining from the Cold War era. Russia had scientists, labs, and a reputation for technology. Education had been one of the top priorities of the Communist regime. Besides, Aziz had felt close to left-wing political thought since his school years. A cadaveric kidney transplanted in Moscow would be a practical and ethical solution to all his concerns. But most important of all, he would not risk the life of a living donor, like he would if he chose to go to India.

Aziz's friend from work who had the transplant in Moscow died some time after the operation due to a heart attack unrelated to his kidney failure. This friend used to work as a tourist guide for a small travel agency, and the agency had taken him to Russia for a transplant when he got sick. In time, as this person realized how profitable a business it would be, his family opened a second office in Istanbul dedicated solely to "transplant tourism" between Moscow and Istanbul. The company required upfront payment in cash for the treatment, the kidney, the flight, and accommodation expenses. One could only hope it remained faithful to its contract, which was a gamble in Turkey. Aziz had good luck. He was in the company of someone who worked as a translator and driver—who not only brought him from the airport to the hospital but also stayed at his service all day for grocery shopping and other needs.

The hospital was a place in transition. Aziz believed that physicians working in the transplant units in Moscow must have been receiving bribes to provide kidneys to foreign recipients like him. How else would all these people get kidneys within a few weeks of hospitalization while under normal circumstances one had to wait for years? The hospital was being updated, renovated, and refurbished, as were many buildings and structures in Moscow. This change must have given him the feeling that the social life of physicians was changing as well.

Aziz was the only Turk who could speak in English to the physicians, the one language they shared. Besides, because of the social distance between the patient and the doctor, most patients, Turkish or Russian, did not dare ask any questions. After his operation, physicians wanted to tell Aziz the identity of his donor. But what good would this do? How would knowing about "a dead Russian" help him? He did not want to know things that had no practical value, yet he speculated it was a female kidney because it atrophied after the transplant. He even joked from time to time that he had a Russian woman inside him. But this was all that he could interpret. He returned from Moscow, continued his career in his company, kept contact with his transplant friends from Russia, and hoped that he could go on with his life as a normal person. He had become healthy again, and this was, like Moscow's future, a promising thing.

CLOSE TO DEATH

I met these patients throughout my fieldwork years and learned from them what it meant to live in a transplanted body and with a sense of self that was changed after the organ transplant. Patients felt reinvented through technology to overcome death. Theirs was an experience intimate with biomedical technological life. Their human condition was the result of many relations hidden and unrevealed, coexisting far from sight. I began thinking about their experiences by looking into the cultures of life and death in which their lives primarily were being shaped. From there, following their pain, suffering, worries, vows, wordings, physicians, travel routes, hospitals, and many other things that seemed essential to them, I tried to understand where their human condition was made meaningful, and how it became theirs to identify with. In their lives in the *biopolis*, I would find the elements by which technology was made into a psychological process. I began to think that their new inner worlds and their transforming boundaries were only reflections of larger social and political changes that could come about through translations, reinventions, imaginaries, myths, and legends.

Sedat, Aziz's hospital friend in Moscow, had repeatedly spoken of how he became a tyrant at home toward his family, especially toward his wife, during his life on dialysis and with her kidney. It was not like him, he said, to be so aggressive and despotic; he could hardly recognize himself in retrospect. Zehra and Oğuz, who received kidneys from their fathers, felt an even deeper change. They began identifying with powerful things that existed beyond their own place in social life such as a *dede* or a robot. Aziz and Fidan remembered the overwhelming physical intensity as they began traveling in their ailing bodies in search of a kidney, and Hatice could not but see her baby, the earthquake, and the lost kidney as parts of one and the same thing: her share from the collective destiny, her *nasib*.

Destiny was one way of dealing with the loss whereas mourning the loss of a kidney was an experience deeply felt by all. Besides, they all seemed to have an unusual feeling for their natural and social environments and their own places in them—something I understood as the emergence of a feeling for the truth within their individual lives resembling an explosion. Zehra's was the most obvious. She lived in an indefinable universe as things from her dreams appeared in the material world and real things began morphing. Fearing death, she began seeing things that she used to think of as imaginary. She began questioning her religious affiliation, her life here-after, her God. She questioned all of these because her family did not refer to Alevi faith in family conversations, and because of the *possibility* of a false path this silence represented. Political problems that used to seem distant to her own well-being, her future, and her place in God's heaven became a fact of her new reality, just as her illness was. She had begun a new social life that was dominated by a nature that had begun moving against its own laws; it was as if something behind the veil of nature were expressing its true face to her.

Any oppression that had a semantic or genealogical relevance to the individual lives of these patients became analogous to their suffering. Fidan could give meaning to her dialysis torture only in terms of her oppression because of her headscarf, which, she believed, felt similar to the invasive routines of the dialysis machine. She believed that the machine, like the headscarf, excluded her from full sociality and from full personhood even though she was a full person with rights. Health care in public institutions was a similar oppression, as inequalities constituted a gap between herself and the state. Besides, modern Turkish history stood between her and medicine that she believed was a product of lies and inventions. She could hardly trust the state's institutions, which had banned her from public education because of her headscarf, and yet she was dependent upon the same public institutions for her recovery from renal failure. It was exactly this kind of terror inherent in the fear of a physical dependency on a machine, on the state, on an artificial system, the fear of something grander and more powerful than the frail human flesh and soul that was forcing many others to find a kidney. That was why it had even crossed her mind to buy a kidney, to cross that line between the humane and the uncivil so that she could liberate herself from dialysis. But something held her back and she waited like many others.

Fidan's feelings of oppression at the dialysis machine were common. Oğuz, in contrast, was a rare case. He preferred to live "like a robot" at the dialysis machine. Instead of a life with his father's kidney, which had somehow rematerialized the troubled relationship between the two within Oğuz's body, he wanted to stay on dialysis and be free of this past. After the transplant he could no longer recognize himself in the mirror. Something within was spoiling his individuality, his features, his hygiene; it was as if something was taking him back to the ocean of life where he was no longer a separate individual. To escape a total loss of himself, Oğuz had found refuge in the robot imagery of life on dialysis, and he had once attempted suicide. To him, like so many others such as Sedat, suicide was a way out of the project "life" that he could no longer deliver.

Aziz was probably the strongest among all of these patients, or maybe this was the impression I had since he had been back to work for a long time already and seemed to be at ease with his life before, during, and after the transplant despite his pain. His financial circumstances, education, and relations had made it easier for him to know the differences between dialysis systems, to travel abroad for a checkup, to be able to talk to physicians with his language skills, to think of the "ethical" solution in finding a kidney, to adapt to life in Moscow, and even to be able to joke about the Russian woman (the transplant) inside him. From Dr. S. of the organ mafia to Dr. Haberal, the founder of transplants in Turkey, Aziz had met many physicians in order to make an informed decision. As I followed his narrative through the cultural aesthetics of transplants in Turkey, I realized in time that his experiences moved through a variety of economic worlds that most patients knew only slightly because of their restricted incomes. Among the wealthy all around the world, however, there were many like Aziz who had become "buyers" in the international networks of trade as travelers in an emerging health tourism related to biotechnological progress.

Through the transplants, patients were stepping into distant hegemonies of medical knowledge, political struggles, idealistic surgeons, the "organ mafia," marginalized and traded bodies, and ideals of technological progress as well as suicides and sacrifice, where *akl-ı selim* (common sense) could not cope. Under an unusual combination of realities, they had to reinvent their uncertain lives as new and proper. As they entered an unusual world, they expected the transplant experience to result in healing and normalcy. Yet, there was no linear change: they did not open one door and enter another familiar reality. Nor was their passage from one simple state or status to another marked by a beginning and an end, or by rites of passage and rituals of closure. They moved instead in a time and space that spiraled without closure, leading them to an altered sense of environment. They encountered unexpected emotions and affectual relations to technology, new selves, new identities. They entered into a new city of meanings, an unfinished biopolis into which they were simultaneously being inducted and constructed.

To understand the foundations of this half-constructed world, I tried to follow them out as far as I could into the cultural and social meanings that my interviewees related. I followed these from fears about an unscrupulous organ mafia to a transplant physician nominated as presidential candidate, from the poor public hospitals to the fancy private ones, from cemeteries to dissection rooms, from suicides to deaths with sacrificial meanings. I wanted to know how people invented and lived through new worlds of life and death, how they experienced new technological objects that already had names and meanings, and how past cultural foundations interacted with the new human condition made possible by biomedical technologies. Over time during my fieldwork, transplantation technology became only one slice of multifaceted social and cultural experiences as was the case for the lives of transplant patients. Dimensions of new lives unfolded for me as I looked into how people and objects were culturally related, how these relationships changed, and how distant worlds became suddenly personal and intimate.

INTERNAL OBJECTS

Following the diagnosis by physicians, patients have spoken to me of medical treatments as having three stages: the renal failure, the dialysis machine, and the transplant. At each stage they would enter another reality and a different psychological process or dynamic: mourning the loss of a kidney; borderline psychosis with dependency on the machine during dialysis; and neurosis triggered by the received kidney and the idea of coming "back to life."

It seemed as if the three different psychic economies caused them to recognize a side of themselves as a bent and misshapen reflection of their earlier selves. They needed readjustment, repairing, reconstruction. These dense experiences were both within and without: the new kidney was not merely a biologically lively organ like other internal organs; it also reorganized social relations that had taken decades to develop. Because of this *tour de corps* they no longer felt safe, private, exclusive, or in control of their own selves. Norms, values, rules of social life seemed radically different now. To understand the newly appearing *unknown* reality and to create a new center in it for themselves, transplant patients needed to develop new life strategies, each doing so individually according to his or her unique past and personhood.

This intimate "politics of life" was driven by mixed feelings toward transplant technology. Neither the dialysis machine nor the transplanted kidney were simple objects of desire. On the contrary, they entered patients' lives abruptly through analogies, such as the headscarf and the oppressive routines of the dialysis machine, only to literally impose a new life upon the world they used to know. Patients would wake up from a coma to find themselves attached to a machine and being told that they would have to learn to live with renal failure. This imposition evoked other oppressive elements. In the aftermath of the operation, as the kidneys physically became parts of their bodies, other emotions came forefront and initiated other awakenings. Things began changing their colors, values, and names. Through the changing nature of things before and after the transplant, patients were confronted with the symbolics of the dialysis machine and the kidney, which echoed a politically unstable world tainted by civil unrest, poverty, and inequality and were reinforced by frightening days spent in hospital corridors and encounters with authoritarian physicians.

Patients described these new realities to me in stories about situations they had encountered throughout the transplant process. They spoke of how they handled organ failure, dialysis routines, the side effects of medications, family dramas, and social pressures of survival. They had to make *lives* their own again but this time through unfamiliar situations with unexpected emotional affects.

To psychoanalysts our mind is constituted by objects that we make our own to be able to relate to the outside world. This process, called introjection, creates internal objects with "good" or "bad" qualities, like the "kind" donor or the "oppressive" dialysis machine. Internal objects are like the shadows of external things falling upon the psyche, or like shadow puppets: we think with them, filter our relationships through them; and in the meanings they provide, we construct our personal worlds. They have a permanent place in our minds.

The kidney, in this sense, represents hope, renewal, and liberation from kidney failure and from the mechanistic routines of dialysis. Unlike the kidney's promise of permanence (even if illusionary), the dialysis machine is seen by patients as a kind of a transitional object that let them live but not thrive. Because of its life-extinguishing character it can be considered a negative or bad object. Because of its mechanistic nature it represents the unwilled place of the artificial in their psyches whose cycles and routines became oppressive and from which patients felt urged to seek liberation.

Patients mourned the loss of a kidney, suffered at the dialysis machine, and hoped for a new kidney, and as they did so certain other internal objects became significant in the interpretation of their lives: the *dede*, the robot, foreign lands, the earthquake, the headscarf, or the experiment. These objects with deep personal and political meanings threw into question patients' places in social life; they operated like an untold dream yet to be interpreted. Drawing paths from inside their bodies toward zones of social life, patients thought they could speak to me of their new selfhoods by narrating their Kafkaesque life histories. They spoke to me of transplants, of medical things, and of the symbolically condensed. In their enveloped words, I could understand how they felt—morphed through things that, external to their wills, had become a part of them.

WORDS OF LIFE

I tried to understand these condensed worlds as anthropologists have before me: exploring basic forms of exchange, social organization, and rites which are situated in contexts and interpretive processes. Through these cultural forms people begin to articulate how knowledge and experience are transformed in modern society. Bridging and weaving together experience, meaning, and existence is central to this cultural work of interpretation. As such, when medical anthropology and medical sociology first began exploring the relevance of organ transplantation to cultural unfoldings of a new human condition, a key arena of attention was the "economy of words" utilized by transplant patients and surgeons.

In the United States, transplant discourse adopted the phrase "gift of life." In their book *The Courage to Fail*, Rene Fox and Judith Swazey, who pioneered fieldwork among transplant patients, wanted to understand what kind of a gift the organ was.[9] They turned to Marcel Mauss's early twentieth-century essay *The Gift*, in which Mauss had argued that "gift exchange" served to reaffirm social bonds and interpersonal relationships. Giving and receiving not only reinforced the strength of relationships among groups but inevitably tied the exchanging parties to the spirit of the exchanged objects; a sense of obligation to reciprocate, which was usually beyond mere equivalence of value, governed the relationship between the recipient and the donor.[10]

The *nature* of these bonds in other words exceeded the object itself. For the Maori, for example, each given individual object was called a *taonga*. It had a spirit, a kind of ethereal life-force, called its *hau* that was as well given away together with the gift. One could utilize the power of the *hau* to evoke and activate *mana*, the magical, spiritual, and religious powers of the collective:

> What imposes obligation in the present received and exchanged, is the fact that the thing received is not inactive. Even when it has been abandoned by the giver, it still posseses something of him. Through it the giver has a hold over the beneficiary just as, being its owner, through it he has a holder over the thief. This is because the *toanga* is animated by the *hau* of its forest, its native heath and soil. It is truly native: the *hau* follows after anyway possesing the things. . . . In reality it is the *hau* that wishes to return to its birthplace, to the sanctuary of the forest and the clan, and to the owner. The *toanga*, or its *hau*—which itself moreover posseses an individuality—is attached to this chain of users.[11]

The gift, then, was like a totem: it accumulated the spirit of the many things it encountered, which expanded with the exchange. Nature, the *mana*, and the former owner all have contributed a life to it. One's power expanded with both the giving and receiving of the gift. The gift, in a way, bore a dangerous relationship.[12]

Just as the spirit embedded in the exchanged object had a unique relationship to its giver, the transplantation of a kidney from one body to

another evoked an altered sense of being for both parties. In organ donation as gift exchange, the donor gave life to the recipient, a gift that could
never be repaid by the recipient: neither an equal exchange nor an exit from
the relation of obligation seemed possible in the experience of transplantation. Organ recipients were enchained in a "tyrannical" social relationship.
The transplanted kidney entered the donor's inner life along with a sense
of dependency and a set of obligations that were hard to return, hard to
pay back, which Fox and Swazey called the "tyranny of the gift."[13] In an
attempt to cover this powerful sense of indebtedness, particularly in the
extreme case of heart donation, American medical practice instituted rules
of anonymity of the donor. In the case of living-related donors of kidneys,
the social ties of extreme giving remained.

Unlike in North America, however, in Turkey renal transplants were not
viewed and discussed using the metaphor of the "gift of life."[14] Transplant
discourse employed the word *bağış*, as in *organ bağışı*, which is translated
as organ donation. The word *bağış* (donation) referred originally to salvation from sin through sacrifice; for example, *kurban bağışı* is the practice of
offering an animal sacrifice following the model or mythic charter of the
Qur'anic story of the sacrifice of İsmail by İbrahim (or of Isaac and Abra-
ham in the Jewish and Christian Bibles). These semantic references are
deeply rooted in the religious references of collective life. *Bağış* also means
a charitable gift. *Organ bağışı* (organ donation) thus echoes the more traditional *kurban bağışı* (sacrificial offering), a sacrificial ritual in which the
body, in parts and pieces, was drawn into an intermediary world. Maybe
because of this sacrificial ritualistic meaning echoing in the medical term
organ bağışı, it has not become as much of an iconic phrase as the English
"gift of life." The effort to introduce a more literal translation from the English "gift of life" as *hayata bağış* did not seem to operate as powerfully as
the English phrase does.[15]

Words referring to life seemed to weigh heavily on transplant patients
when I talked to them. In general they remained silent where normally
one might use the words *death* or *life* in connection with donors. Yet, the
Turkish language richly utilizes varieties of the words "life" and "death" and
there were many efforts to utilize new words for brain death so as not to
confuse it with a vegetative state, or with life.

Jann (written in Turkish as *can*) is the term used most commonly to
refer to life and its vivid liveliness. It is a word originating in Persian and

means life as a metaphysical thing that animates the body. It is akin to the Greek word *zoë*. *Hayat*, from Arabic, is also commonly used to refer to life but more in relation to social energy that keeps people alive and together. Another word, *yaşam*, also means life with an emphasis on life's duration between birth and death, its continuity, and its quality. *Yaşam* is a word used in modern biology. In transplantation discourse, *jann* and *hayat* have a special place and are alternative usages. *Jann*, in social life, is particularly used to refer to a metaphysical entity *given* (*Can vermek*) but never *taken* (*Can almak*). *Can almak* (to take one's life) is used to describe the violation of the right to live. In the everyday language of transplant patients, the metaphysics associated with the word *jann* play a central role regarding the right to give life and the ban against taking it: a brain-dead donor or a living donor who is related to the recipient both give *jann* to the patients in need of kidneys. In both cases, *jann* is given to an ill person after being taken from another, a brain-dead or living donor. Giving and taking life is the language also of crime and innocence and its use in the technology of transplantation creates and fosters a confusion of associated meanings.

The donated kidney is "life saving" (*hayat kurtarır*). It gives *jann*—a rough analog of the Maori *hau*[16]—to the ailing body of a patient. In the metaphysical act of becoming alive again, the donor and the recipient are both subsumed under the organ's depersonalized yet collective *jann*. For this reason, the act of donation does not imply giving a "gift of life" in which the gift is viewed as a Cartesian spare part by the medical community. Rather *jann* is the metaphysical entity that animates the *emanet*, the body entrusted from God to the human being for safe keeping; and in transplants, the *jann* of a donated kidney from an *emanet* body animates the patient's depleted body to keep it alive.

As the stages of the transplant proceed, many corners of culture concerning the body, ownership, privacy, and the divine are activated in emotion-laden words and phrases. Some of the deployed words are traditional and some are recently invented, some "work" to achieve technological ends and some do not. As time passes, patients internalize a variety of these words and associations, along with worries embedded in them, as well as other personal histories and meanings, which become part of the always unfinished worlds they build and inhabit. I began interpreting these unfinished technological lives in hospital rooms where political fights and institutional tensions were staged in the name of saving patients' lives. There, patients were diagnosed with renal failure, sent to dialysis, prescribed medications, operated upon, and treated for the rest of their lives with immunosuppressants, occasional dialysis, and further transplants. There, in hospital rooms, patients found a new kind of family with an unusual and *unknown* history into which somehow they had to fit.

THE BIOPOLIS

Transplantation is a deeply problematic practice as transplant physicians have repeated over the years. I met surgeons, nephrologists, ICU physicians, transplant physicians, nurses, and heads of many transplant units in Istanbul, Ankara, and Antalya as I began mapping a topography of this highly politicized medical practice. From them, I learned that the practice of transplantation was mainly split between opposing ideas about life and death, about how to treat and value the "cadaver" and the "brain-dead" donor, about how to make use of the *jann*, and about how to explain and relate this use value of death and *jann* to the public.

Most of the transplanted kidneys were harvested from living donors in Turkey. Physicians would frequently compare their donor pools and infrastructure to those of other European countries and complain that European rates of cadaveric transplants were much higher than in Turkey. The European Union averaged 15 to 30 brain-dead donors per million population, with Spain scoring the highest rate of 50 brain-dead donors per million, whereas in Turkey this ratio was less than 2.4 brain-dead donors per million.[17] The dramatic difference represented the outlook toward death, life, and a cultural relationship with the divine, which, physicians thought, in a mysterious way, determined the inner workings of the transplant economy.

Almost all physicians agreed that Turkish people's anxieties about mutilation of the dead body, fears of purgatory because of having violated the body borrowed from God, or other religious concerns were the root cause of the difficulty in obtaining brain-dead donors for transplants. Culture stood between physicians and donors. It was a domain that physicians were reluctant to enter, and when they did so it was with much navigation and with the support of publicly acknowledged authorities in religion and the media. If the issue was something physicians assumed would not raise much public reaction, then they thought of it as a "possible" domain where medicine could be practiced. If, in contrast, it would be a scandal, then they tried to find ways through institutional and hegemonic structures to make the "impossible" possible. As a result, a discourse on the "possible" versus the "impossible" was born in transplant units to justify and legitimize desirable biopolitical agendas and to make technology reach its progressive ends, this time inside the body.

Their discourse was reminiscent of that of space exploration with its utopian and dark sides. Sputnik went up in the late 1950s, sparking a scientific and military race between the United States and the Union of Soviet Socialist Republics. The first heart transplant occurred a decade later, triggering a stop-and-go set of advances and failures in transplant technologies and a debate about the emergence of black markets and inequalities of access to good healthcare. Turkish transplant practice began around the same time as space research in the United States and the Soviet Union, the military action of 1971 in Turkey that had the impact of a coup, the global oil crises of 1974, and student movements throughout the 1970s. It was an invisible biopolis unseen under their shadows at first.

In 1969, in the wake of the first human-to-human heart transplant, which was performed in South Africa in 1967 by Christian Bernard, Turkish surgeons in Istanbul conducted two heart transplants, both of which resulted in failure. Many physicians ignored this beginning as they told me of the history of transplants in Turkey, but others saw it as essential in understanding Turkish physicians' attitudes toward transplants. One transplant surgeon admired the courage of physicians at that time. To him, these operations should be recognized as the first transplants in the country because they showed the courage of Turkish physicians and their ability to conduct such high-tech operations at such an early time. Moreover, he, like many other physicians, saw transplant technology as analogous to space exploration; as such, losing a few space shuttles, he said, should be considered "normal" in the early stages of such a high profile practice.

In the early 1970s a team of surgeons at Hacettepe (Ankara University Medical School) headed by Dr. Mehmed Haberal began experimental studies on liver transplantation.[18] The first successful transplant in Turkey was a kidney transplant from a living-related donor conducted at Hacettepe in 1975 by this team.[19] In 1978 the same group successfully transplanted a cadaveric kidney provided by the Eurotransplant organ allocation network. Despite the successful operation, physicians thought that Turkey was not yet ready to integrate local brain-dead bodies into its technological transformation at that time. The insufficient infrastructure from dialysis machines to respirators was a pending problem. For this reason patients like Sedat were encouraged to go to the United Kingdom when they needed transplants. In the meantime, physicians kept thinking of obtaining brain-dead donors; they even received kidneys from Germany and other European countries with the help of Eurotransplant.[20] At Hacettepe, they worked steadily to provide sufficient technological infrastructure for transplantation, draft regulatory legislation, inform the public about transplantation, initiate dialysis programs for patients with renal failure, improve access to immunosuppressive drugs, educate medical staff, improve tissue typing, graft imaging, and immunosuppressive drug monitoring, and collaborate with European physicians and organ-sharing networks.[21]

Haberal believed that of all these technical and organizational efforts the most essential and immediate one was to form a bond between medicine and the public. Physicians had to provide the public with an image of transplantation that would help create a donor pool from brain-dead donors or living bodies if their work was to be a legitimate biomedical practice rather than a project.

Along with Haberal, the biopolis began appearing in the visions of two other surgeons from Hacettepe: Dr. Tuncer Karpuzoğlu and Dr. Münci Kalayoğlu. All three had close contacts with transplant teams in the United States, all three had friends at the Grand National Assembly of Turkey at the time, and all three viewed transplantation as Turkey's most prestigious high-tech practice. In their hands, they dreamed back then, Turkey could become a world leader in surgery and scientific practice.

Their visions materialized as the world economy slowly began changing. With the support of Turgut Özal, then the prime minister, Karpuzoğlu helped establish the Akdeniz University Medical School and its transplant unit in Antalya.[22] In 1982, Kalayoğlu left for the United States to become a world-class transplant surgeon at the University of Wisconsin, Madison. A few years later, Haberal founded the Middle East Society for Organ Transplants (MESOT, 1987), the Turkish Transplantation Society (TOD, 1990), and Başkent University in Ankara (1991). As these universities, foundations, and societies were established, surgeons became more independent to make decisions in favor of transplants' infrastructure and legislation.

Unlike the developments in Ankara and Antalya that favored semi-private and private health care, in Istanbul transplantation initiatives took on a more socialist vision of medicine in the early 1990s. Working from Çapa (Istanbul University Medical School Hospital), Dr. Uluğ Eldegez, who had returned from his internship in Essen, Germany, founded an NGO that launched a regional organ-sharing database dedicated solely to transplants from brain-dead donors. Eldegez was concerned about transplanting organs from living-related donors because doctors could not trust or police the claims of living-related donors to be legitimate members of the three legal categories for donation: he was worried about organ trafficking.[23] He had seen the success of transplant teams in Essen in obtaining brain-dead donors and in being able to maintain an efficient practice with such donations. He decided to establish a transplant unit to pioneer "cadaveric" transplants. In time, his unit's efforts to transplant organs from brain-dead bodies under the poor conditions in a public hospital made him an icon of idealistic transplant medicine. Many physicians in the younger generation looked up to his efforts to overcome the taboos surrounding the dead body within medicine.

Throughout the 1990s there was tension between Ankara and Istanbul; neither of the centers acknowledged each other's practice. This resulted in dual organ allocation databases, foundations, and international representation as well as separate donor pools nationwide. In the same years the idea of an organ mafia, too, became publicly propagated by the media. By the beginning of the 2000s, the Ministry of Health, which many believed to have only a symbolic role in the organization of transplants up to that point, drafted legislation for transplantation regulations that was suited to the economic boom that had transformed Turkish medicine so radically since 1989. Bureaucrats tried to unify organ allocation databases and networks, standardize certain diagnostic tools, manage rumors of an organ mafia, and stand over the medical institutions, which were becoming strong, private, and independent. There was an invisible tension between neoliberal market-based medicine and idealistic public hospital physicians, and between private hospitals and public ones, just as there was a difference of opinion on living-related transplants versus cadaveric transplants. In time, private hospitals multiplied and successfully lobbied the government to allow them to run their own transplant units. By 2003, in new marble, glass, and steel corporate hospital buildings one could pay high sums for a transplant operation. And in 2007, Münci Kalayoğlu, who had been working in the United States since 1981, returned to Turkey to run the transplant unit at Memorial Hospital in Istanbul. For him, as for Eldegez, the issue related to brain death was to improve transplantation nationwide. However, instead of hoping for more donations from the public like Eldegez, Kalayoğlu hoped to improve cadaveric donation rates by changing Turkish physicians' outlooks toward brain death.

Biopolis was no longer a vision. It had materialized as an economic universe of biological objects, a reflection of a variety of political agendas, a domain of possibilities. Having become a slice of the cultural universe, in Turkey it was born into a unique local history as well. Turkey's past resembled a parallel universe caught between continents, languages, and peoples, which had to be reinvented to host the modern self with its cultural and technical infrastructures. Turkey's modernity and its passions were guarding the body in many ways. Somewhere between the East and the West, the country was a synthetic space, a continuum of meaning. Patients were learning to fit in the biopolis's history as it emerged from their country's political past with its myths, legends, and stories that were partly *known* to them from their family histories.

EAST OF "REASON," WEST OF "ETERNAL LIFE"

In a short passage in his novel *Tanyeri Horozları* (2002), Yaşar Kemal depicts the beginnings of democratic life in the young Turkish republic. He tells us the story of people of diverse ethnic origins—Kurds, Turks, Greeks, Laz, and Çerkez—who left their homes to fight for the Ottoman Empire in World War I and then with Atatürk in the Turkish War of Independence. In the years of fighting, these people, like my ancestors, lost almost everything they had: their villages were burned; their families scattered and lost. Personifications of the nation's tragic history, Kemal's characters found their way to a small, deserted island off the Aegean coast of Anatolia where they could start a new life in a peaceful environment surrounded by the milky waters of the island's shoreline and the perfumed air from Mount Ida filling their mornings. These were people who used to be inhabitants of a large and heterogeneous empire. Their occupations were as diverse as their ethnic and religious origins. In a way, these differences, which could be a problem in other times, made it easy enough for them to return to an efficient life given the diversity of their occupations and skills. In a time of transition, it bonded them with an unusual sense of community—that is, as Kemal depicts, until the first politician came to town to deliver a propaganda speech on the new regime. Little did they know how politics in the new regime had changed, and how the magical things that inhibited their tales would take on new lives even before they themselves took on new lives:

> This nation is the Anka Kuşu [the phoenix]. The Anka Kuşu is the king of all birds; it lives one thousand years, and then a fire shines from its chest. The Anka Kuşu burns to ashes with this fire, a single egg is born out of its ashes, a warm newborn hatches from this egg, the newborn grows up in seven days, [and it] becomes the king of all birds. And in this way the Anka Kuşu lives majestically until Kıyamet [the Day of Judgment] comes. Our ancestors, our race are the Anka Kuşu of all humankind. Like the egg born out of ashes, we will also be reborn until the Day of Judgment comes. Our ancestors and our republic will live forever through Mustafa Kemal Atatürk. My victorious people, today I have come here to open the People's Republican Party.[24]

Kemal's novel depicted the top-down transition from traditional life to modernity, from ethnic and religious diversity to a unified nation-state, and from an Oriental worldview to an Occidental one. The Anka Kuşu was reintroduced as the symbol of hope as these transitions to an uncertain future took place. It was hoped to ease people into the new rhetoric.

Traditionally, wherever the Anka Kuşu landed, new tales began. I, like everyone else, grew up hearing stories about its travels. It is no wonder that in Kemal's depiction the beginning of Turkey's political life and the birth of the modern democratic regime in the republican era were initiated by it because it was like the beginnings of those tales. It was born of death and ashes; it was new again. Similarly, as suggested by the terms "Young Ottomans" and "Young Turks"—the famous names given to the nationalists and modernizers who brought the republic into being—there was a constant feeling of excitement and youth embodied in all matters regarding modernity and its discontents that was represented in participation in political life, being the subject of a sovereign state, and living through discoveries and technologies. People seemed to be forever conscious of this youthfulness.

Anka represented the strength of this youth and flew through the big and ever changing structures of modernity to ease people's everyday struggles and to help them maintain normal lives in the face of the radical unexpected social and political changes. Modernity was impressively grand: it was making things proper, creating an order equivalent to that in the "civilized" world of the West, which had been inspired by universal and humanistic values. When, despite all efforts, things did not happen in modern Turkish life as they do in Western models, people felt vulnerable and oppressed by it. The Anka Kuşu flapped its wings and flew through it to make order from disorder, to become Occidental, to prove the value of ever increasing knowledge of the material world. It was transforming the legendary souls and their afterlives as told in tales for the sake of the continuity of community, the family, and the self. Modernity transformed the self like this through meta-political histories: it was a top-down change. Local cultures were romanticized and utilized to provide deep emotions for the land and the ancestors.

The Turkish republic was founded in 1923. But the rise of medicine and people's place in the grand structure of life, which was slowly manifesting itself, had begun much earlier in 1789.

For Ottomans, the significance of the French Revolution far exceeded the images of the riots, the guillotine, the blood streaming through the streets of Paris, and the vengeful poor of the Reign of Terror in 1793–94. Influenced by the dramatic effects of the French Revolution, from 1789 to 1807 Selim III, the Ottoman sultan, attempted to implement a set of reforms called the New Order (Nizam-ı Cedid). He was overthrown, however, by the Yeniçeris (Janissaries, the sultan's bodyguard corps) whom he wanted to abolish to modernize the military. In 1826, his successor, Mahmud II, succeeded against the old Janissary institution and launched a new era to establish modern institutions that would become centers of modern life in the Turkish republic later on. Both the newly founded Tıbhane, the medical school (1827), and the Kara Harp Okulu, the Turkish Military Academy (1834), were the pioneering steps into a modern technological life.

The Tanzimat (Reorganization) Era (1839–76) followed these. It was the most eventful reform period of the nineteenth century, especially with regard to the invention of the subject and the introduction of individual liberties. It began with the edict Gülhane Hatt-ı Hümayun in 1839 as the new sultan, Abdülmecid I, granted equal rights to all subjects of the empire. The

Meclis-i Maarif-i Umumiye, an early form of the first Ottoman Parliament (1876), was established in 1848 after the edict. At a time when in Europe Wolfgang von Kempelen's chess-playing automaton "the Turk" was being displayed in European courts and fairs, the Turkish sultans were building a modern state and establishing a parliament, fighting domestic corruption, establishing national academies, and laying the foundations for a national life for which the subject would become the citizen. "The Turk" won at chess as it traveled across Europe and overseas, while the Ottomans actually knew they were losing.

With these reforms, the people of the Ottoman Empire were transformed from a mass to be governed by the Sultan into a public with representation. As the era progressed, public intellectuals, writers, and poets emerged and gave voice to the individual as a bearer of rights. One of the most prominent among them was Namık Kemal (1840–88), a writer for the Ottoman paper *Tasvir-i Efkar*. Kemal was a founding member of the Young Turk movement and a key reformer of Turkish thought who introduced ideas of freedom and patriotism into Ottoman public life.[25] Inspired by Kemal and others, the Young Turk reform movement had a profound impact on the intellectual environment of the time. The Young Turks expressed their radical views in newspapers and poetry. Beginning in the late 1880s these people opened an era of criticism of the machinery of social life. Their idea was to change the imperial regime.

Mustafa Kemal Atatürk, a young soldier and war hero in the Ottoman army in those years, was influenced by Namık Kemal's ideas on freedom. In 1919, soon after the German and Ottoman defeat at the end of World War I, Mustafa Kemal took control of the Ottoman military forces,[26] declared a war of independence, and founded the modern Turkish parliament. The new parliament strived not only to reform the political structure of the country by abolishing the sultanate, but also to liberate itself from foreign occupation and ensure national autonomy for the people of Anatolia. The war ended with the Conference of Lausanne in 1923, which established the new nation's borders, defined its population, and changed its name from the Ottoman Empire to the Republic of Turkey.

With the fall of the empire came the birth of the republic upon the reformist values and institutions that had been established in the empire over the previous one hundred years. The republic embraced the values of universal equality, humanism, and enlightenment that had been embraced by the Young Turk movement and its precursors. It was liberated from both Ottoman rule and the Western occupiers. In this sense Kemalism tried to balance the loss of rulers as both sovereigns and oppressors with the invention of a modernity based on universal values and ideals of progress. Kemalism looked into the future to materialize ideals of equality, secularism, nationalism, and sovereignty.

The youthfulness of this beginning underlined the national ethos, as the new regime, the political party, and institutions depicted in Kemal's novel exemplify. In the big cities, a national symphony, ballets, theaters, dams, factories, and schools were built in the spirit of this youth.[27] In 1924, the republic abolished the caliphate as well as powerful Islamic institutions. Other reforms followed. Words themselves changed as the republic adopted the Latin alphabet instead of the Arabic script. This reform, in combination with the ban of the fez—the official trademark of modern Ottoman bureaucrats—and the veil and all religious symbols from public life, constituted the strongest gesture of resistance against the patriarchal structures of the old imperial Ottoman rule. The fez, the veil, the beard, the dancing forms of the Arabic alphabet, and the mystic sects were the ashes of an era that had to vanish for the new beginning to unfold. And dialectically, in time these symbols would form the basis of the opposition to the new regime.

First, people began looking different. Unlike the gradual transitions of the nineteenth-century reforms, change came rapidly in the new era. With the ban on the veil and fez, Turks were expected to dress in the latest Western fashions. Today's Turkish republican elite still dresses in the Western style, in contrast to the increasingly popular recent adaptation by women of the turban and the headscarf. With the new republic, people moved from one way of being in the world into another, and this dramatic political superimposition affected their self-knowledge. Illustrations of how to dress, talk, and walk "properly" decorated the public imaginary. Among the elites, one had to consult books, go to schools, and read and write with the "proper" language to ensure one's place in the social hierarchy of the modern world, as was the case in the West. The new image of the country, which was centered on nation building, destabilized traditional self-conceptions this way.

Like one invents names for objects to make them one's own, one always invents spaces to be able to host things. In this sense the geographical space was reinvented to make it Turkey's. To this end, the Ministry of Education began publishing books on an Anatolian cultural heritage that belonged just to Turkey. Because Mustafa Kemal could not draw on Ottoman identity or Islam as anchorage points, he turned to ancient cultures as was fashionable in the first half of the twentieth century.[28] The new republic was almost 15 percent of the size of the old Ottoman Empire, yet the breadth and depth of its tales increased as the prehistoric peoples of Anatolia were added to the official history of the nation, supplying a cultural and historical density that compensated for the geophysical loss. This new history of the people was carved by the depth of time upon the republic's precious geographic space. It was a eugenicist project of the sort common in the early twentieth century: as always, tales mingled with genealogies to invent people through noble kinship ties, only this time they did so under the systematic production of the state and its selection processes.[29]

People were like clay in the hands of a state, which had invented the nation and then began molding its subjects where the Ottoman reformations had left off. Yet, different from those early reform periods in the nineteenth century, cultural reformation lay at the heart of the republic's nation building.[30] Along with industrialization, this change came to bear the politics of self-knowledge, the cultural inheritance of the past, and the possibilities of the future. In time, a separation of the old ways from the new through an analogy of legends and political action was beginning to define a Turkish identity into which transplant patients were born.

In history and ethnography, Turks had found a virtual path back to ancestors who had been lost over centuries. The Turkish tribes of Central Asia that had moved west during a long period of migration throughout the first millennium were one such link. The Oğuz tribe, to which the Ottoman family belonged, had begun its westward journey about the tenth century. The Oğuz's legends, myths, and shamanic symbols such as the horse, the tree, and the gray wolf, along with the Hittite sun of central Anatolia, and the Simurg of Persian myths, became imaginary beings bonding Turks to a long past and a distant wide space. The institutionalization of legends and myths as national culture transformed old symbols into transcendental political objects; it distanced them from their previous role as immanent elements of technologies of the self.[31] To teach people to become subjects of a nation, powerful and magical symbols were incorporated into politics and national history in ways in which people could relate from oral folk traditions. This allowed rich and dense time and space for communal life.[32]

At the same time, the orthodoxy of Sunni Islam was appropriated. The republic established the Diyanet (Presidency of Religious Affairs), and gave it the authority to govern the religious life in the country. In time political parties would both control and utilize orthodox religious and mythic nationalist symbolism to mobilize people for political ends. While some of the symbols were institutionalized, struggles of everyday life were poeticized, glorified, and turned into social codes by poets and public intellectuals. The tension between the realms of the everyday and the official attested to people's ability to create a space for personal reflection, growth, and love in the midst of repression and political chaos—a space that would coexist alongside the biopolis in patients' and physicians' worlds.

In many ways, Turkish people were a great example of the execution of modernity upon a population that had become members of a young nation. In the first half of the twentieth century, under the leadership of Mustafa Kemal, this young national identity was invented through reforms that began population counts (1927), abolished Islam as the state religion (1928), granted women the right to vote (1930), initiated surnames (1934), and allowed five-time daily prayers to be conducted in Turkish instead of Arabic (1941). At the same time, the young nation also tried to find a balance between the rising National Socialism in Germany and the Soviet presence in the north.

Mustafa Kemal died in 1938 before the Second World War. İsmet İnönü, his right hand in the war of independence, became the next president. During the Second World War Turkey had declared neutrality and kept it almost until the end of the war when it finally joined the Allies. The CHP was a strong defender of Kemalist values. It won the first multiparty elections that took place in 1946 but lost the next elections against the conservative Demokrat Parti (DP) led by Adnan Menderes.[33] The DP's line was close to the United States. It was populist. It had made peace with Turkey's Ottoman Muslim heritage—a line unacceptable to the new republic.[34] Turkey's troubling years of social violence would also begin in the aftermath of the DP's rule in 1960 as students began clashing at universities, curfews were imposed, and a coup d'état followed. As the military took over control of the country and ruled it with a temporary cabinet, Milli Birlik Komitesi (MBK), it drafted a civil constitution, banned the DP from political life, and hanged its leaders in 1961. This was how political upheavals throughout the country, especially at the universities, had begun. Students, workers, Communists, Muslims, and nationalists each had established different groups in search of stable political identity, justice, and equality. The opposing ideologies of the two Cold War masters—the neighboring Soviet Union in the north and the "defender of the free world," the United States, to the west—were the two main opposing political platforms in Turkey, where the political consciousness was staged, yet there was much fragmentation between these two poles too. In the streets, though, violence had taken over, as the CHP went into coalition with the right-wing Adalet Partisi (AP), headed by Necmettin Erbakan, the first politician of the republic to defend Islam as a model for political governance.[35]

Throughout the 1970s, student organizations were banned, intellectuals and academics attacked, columnists murdered. And as the turmoil in the Middle East and Turkey peaked, communes of left-wing youth expressed their desire to empower people. At times they invoked the spirit of the poet Nâzım Hikmet, who, during exile in Bulgaria in 1957, had penned the poem "Ceviz Ağacı" (The walnut tree) as a tribute to the ideals of the Gülhane Hatt-ı Hümayun.[36] The lyrics had become a left-wing liberation song, among others, invoking the spirit of the poet now living in the metaphoric walnut tree.[37]

> My head is a foaming cloud, inside and outside I'm the sea.
> I am a walnut tree in Gülhane Park in İstanbul,
> an old walnut tree with knots and scars.
> You don't know this and the police don't either.
>
> I am a walnut tree in Gülhane Park.
> My leaves sparkle like fish in water,
> my leaves flutter like silk handkerchiefs,
> Break one off, my darling, and wipe your tears.
> My leaves are my hands—I have a hundred thousand hands.
> İstanbul I touch you with one hundred thousand hands.
> My leaves are my eyes, and I am shocked at what I see.
> I look at you, İstanbul, with a hundred thousand eyes
> And my leaves beat, beat with a hundred thousand hearts.
>
> I am a walnut tree in Gülhane Park.
> You don't know this and the police don't either.[38]

While people tried to continue life as normal, the tension peaked throughout the 1970s as students armed themselves at the universities and medical schools. Some of the physicians I met had studied through these hard years and had been engaged in the left-wing movement. It was in these years that the transplant law was prepared and the first operations were conducted. As gunshots became a natural part of the sounds beginning by sunset in those days, on September 12, 1980, the military took over again. It intervened in the democratic process, jailing many individuals while some intellectuals and academics escaped into exile in Europe. People felt the pressure of a life pushing down from somewhere up above—from the gray sky where heaven was supposed to reside, where angels were supposed to fly, where still, despite everything, the beautiful moon dressed and un-dressed regularly. How could danger and threat be pouring into life when tales and stories, like that of the Anka Kuşu, spoke of a past of kindness and foresaw a future filled with light and hope? These tales were dear because living had become dangerous. Hope and change had become empty words. They were unreal.

In the years that followed the putsch, Turkish transplantation practice began emerging, and in a decade, the world order began changing; and so did political life in Turkey. The PKK (Kurdistan Workers' Party) offi-cially declared war against the Turkish state in 1984, and in 1989 the mili-tary acknowledged this declaration and responded with the declaration of war against terror. Many people had fled the country for Europe and the United States right after the putsch, returning only in the 1990s. In the same era, Kalayoğlu went to the United States to learn transplantation, whereas Haberal was drafting, refining, and adapting the transplant law according to local cultural sensitivities. Amid the putsch and the lack of political diver-sity where former party leaders had been banned from political life, Turgut Özal, who used to work for the IMF and was known as an "Americanist," won the next elections to become the prime minister and later on the next president of the country. Throughout the 1980s and 1990s Turkey went through further turbulence, this time financially, and struggled to come to terms with its oppressed religious and ethnic groups. Özal's relations with the United States and his neoliberal policies had a great impact on the transformation of Turkish medicine. While Haberal and Karpuzoğlu could utilize their "own" medical schools, others, who were more interested in a socialist and public vision of medicine, emerged in Istanbul and then in İzmir, Antalya, Bursa, Adana, and a few other cities and networked under separate webs, separate cultures of medicine, separate worldviews. Patients had to make their choices in this fragmented biopolis and its hegemonic political agendas.

REGULATING HUMAN AFFAIRS, FEARS, EMOTIONS

If anything made the deepest impression on me regarding the practice of transplantation, it was the hardships physicians endured in their efforts to make transplantation independent functioning units in their hospitals using an invented language that worked against cultural taboos but with the traditions of medicine and modernity. Physicians had endured poverty, lack of infrastructure, taboos surrounding the dead body, institutional power struggles, and, amid these troubles, the emerging market of organ trading. They faced, internalized, and transformed these difficulties as they expanded their practices over these sub-universes, or slices of lifeworlds, which existed beforehand and intersected with their futures.

Sharing the Dead

Hard days often mark the beginning of one's vocation and dominate one's feeling for it as one grows into it. And so, most of the senior physicians I have known sank into deep thought as they described the circumstances in which transplantation as a practice was born. In 1980, just as the Turkish Transplantation and Burn Foundation was being founded, for example, within a matter of days the military coup of September 12 emptied the streets of protestors and stilled the public life of poets.[39] News of Haberal's transplant unit in those days reflected the dominant poverty and despair throughout the country:

> Suffering patients fill hospital corridors hoping to find imuran[40] or a dialysis machine. It costs 15,000 lira to cleanse one's blood at the kidney [dialysis] machine. The poor are left to die. . . .
>
> The shadow of death has fallen over their [patients'] frozen eyes, and over their yellow texture. . . . They speak with a weak and low tone: "We want to live. We are waiting for kidneys," they say. Another patient asks

with a stronger tone, "Did imuran arrive?" inquiring about the medication. They are protected by their Blue Angels [the surgeons] and the white dressed nurses and doctors who, with God's permission, will heal them.

This is the miserable picture at Hacettepe University Hospital's transplant unit. Our hearts are filled with sorrow, and we talk to [the patients] kindly while we peek at Azrail [the angel of death].[41]

These images of angels, colors, doctors, machines, and drugs evoked feelings of a destitute biomedical suffering, an unbearable human condition that materialized in these bodies in need of transplants. The silenced public must have absorbed the death-loaded news of transplants with impressions of political repression. In this way the rhetoric of organ donation must have entered public life and invaded the private sphere, interfering with the closely guarded secret of personal lives; it was as if the state wanted to extend its hegemony into the intimate domain of the family, as if its technocratic policies were demanding something from within the body to make this possible. In this atmosphere news of transplants and organ donation expressed an aura less of altruism than of an expected civic duty. The media attention to transplantation actually increased in the months following the putsch and continued despite political tension.[42] That same year standardized organ donation cards were printed to introduce the virtues of organ donation to the public.

I was introduced to these beginning years by Haberal when he told me his side of the story. These were days of hard work at Hacettepe as they launched the transplant unit: their initial social challenge was to avoid being misunderstood, to prevent being labeled as "scavengers" who hoped for death in order to profit from it. He did not seem to think highly of the beginning years of transplants anywhere in the world. In the 1960s the dialysis machine was being used to treat chronic kidney failure. Transplantation technology improved after this and in time the number of patients on transplant waiting lists grew with it but the number of donors did not keep that pace. The brain-dead body had become an important source from which to transplant organs and that was why cadaveric transplants were encouraged. He thought it was unfortunate that the number of cadaveric donations in the Middle East and in many developing countries was so low compared to those in Europe and the United States. By the 1970s, for example, in

Europe, 75 percent of all organ transplants were cadaveric whereas in Turkey into the new millennium 80 to 90 percent of all transplants were from living donors. Haberal felt that he and his team pioneered transplants in a country where poverty and the challenges of political life worked against technological progress.

In 1975 at Hacettepe, Haberal and his team had conducted the first successful living-related transplant from a Turkish donor, and a few years later the first cadaveric transplant with a kidney donated from the European organ-sharing network Eurotransplant. But Haberal realized that a few gifts from Eurotransplant would not be enough to establish a routine medical practice. They had to find cadaveric organs locally instead of expecting kidneys from Europe.

Before the putsch in 1980, Haberal had helped draft the informed consent legislation on organ transplantation and tissue grafting that allowed harvesting of organs from living or dead donors. With this law enacted, he would conduct the first domestic cadaveric kidney transplant that same year. Despite the new law, there were very few donations and he still had to rely on Europe. For this reason, his team began conducting experiments to develop a cold ischemia preservation technique that could keep cadaveric kidneys viable for more than one hundred hours following harvesting. This would make it easier to use donated kidneys from Eurotransplant.[43]

In 1982, due to a continuing lack of donations, Haberal proposed a change in legislation. If they had more donations from living bodies, they would be able to conduct more transplants instead of expecting local cadaveric donations or gifts from Eurotransplant. This would also stabilize their donor pool. To pursue this, Haberal proposed a system inspired by regulations in the United States that would permit organ donations from immediate family members as well as more distantly related people.

This new definition proposed three categories of kinship relations that would qualify as living-related organ donors: the first degree of kin pertained to parents and children of a patient; the second degree of kin covered more distant relatives, such as uncles, aunts, and cousins; and the third degree of kin included people who were emotionally attached to the patient even if they were not necessarily biologically related, such as partners, stepchildren, and friends. The third category not only allowed transplant patients to bring along their "loved ones" as donors but, in years to come, it would allow the organ mafia to continue its practice upon a quasi-legal platform. It was from this third-degree kin that transplant patients began informally to purchase organs.[44] Such transactions remained within the realm of legality as long as the donor-sellers signed papers affirming their voluntary participation and physicians did not know of it. I have met many physicians who often in despair complained about the quasi-illegal transplant practices and the law, which allowed the third-degree kinship. With it, they thought, the criminal had emerged, but without it the number of transplants overall would decrease.

"The whole thing is out of control because patients bring their donors, introducing them as their relatives, or they claim the third degree of kinship, the emotional tie. . . . It is difficult to tell who is who. Poverty is the main problem we are facing in Turkey and under these circumstances transplantation regulations are not ethical enough," a young transplant surgeon had told me. By 2000, 80 percent of the donations in Başkent University were from living-related donors. "We do not reject a patient who brings his or her own donor. Actually, in this hospital there is no other way: either you find a donor or we put your name on the list for cadaveric donors. Dr. Haberal does not take care of patients who go to Russia or India to have a transplant and then come back and want to be taken care of. Due to the low donation rates from cadaveric donors, most patients have to bring their own donors unless they want to be listed in the organ-sharing database."

Physicians had differences of opinion on the value of living bodies versus dead ones. The dispute had begun shaping the institutionalization process early on. Eldegez and Haberal had become rivals because of the database, which entailed the characteristic of the donors and was the essential information pool of transplant politics for patients and physicians alike. It began when Eldegez came back from Germany and established a transplant unit dedicated to cadaveric transplants. To do this he needed a nationwide database: he had to network with other hospitals, follow brain death diagnoses, and share information. The database was Eldegez's most ambitious project. It had been one of the original goals of his work since he began in 1991. Yet, Haberal and his team in Ankara, which pioneered transplants, were not eager to become a part of it as they had their own list. Istanbul and Ankara then respectively allied with other hospitals in their regions, which lead to the establishment of two different organ-sharing networks, two different transplant societies, two different approaches to the donor pool, in short two of everything. The database was split geographically, epistemologically, theologically, and so biopolitically.

At Istanbul University Medical School, a nationwide NGO called the Organ Coordination Center was planned to govern the database and to match patients with brain-dead donors in other hospitals. This was the only way to make efficient use of the available brain-dead donors. All transplant teams in Istanbul and elsewhere had to operate with a set of scientific and social protocols for issues like the criteria for diagnosing brain death. But even if all of this worked efficiently, there were other problems stemming from power struggles and differences of opinion, all of which affected the choice of the hospital that would be the "cadaveric" organ's destination. Eldegez explained,

> Turkey is a developing country. We have to make decisions based on population statistics. How many transplants do we do per million people? Austria does thirty, Spain fifty-six, Germany thirty-eight. We should be around 30 but we perform many fewer operations—we do one per million. Our statistical situation is very poor compared to EU countries. We are trying to establish a database here at the coordination center to unite twenty-eight centers in fourteen cities. We are the center of it all. Let me give you an example: if there is a cadaver donor in Adana [a city in the south of Turkey], we can match the tissue and send it to İzmir [a city on the Aegean coast]. The transplant unit in Adana has the right to keep one kidney for its patients. The other kidney is matched in the common database to be sent to [a patient in] another city. We distribute organs according to the norms established by Eurotransplant and United Network for Organ Sharing (UNOS) and not according to "Ottoman mentality."[45]

The Organ Coordination Center, which tried to implement a rational sharing system, operated until 2001 in Istanbul and helped to organize many hospitals in the city and the region. In 2001, the Ministry of Health decided to unify the networks. It transferred full control of the Organ Coordination Center from Istanbul to Ankara, where Haberal was already located. In the meantime, the Turkish economy had begun transforming itself from state control into a neoliberal market. Many private hospitals were founded. Physicians had become mobile in order to work for them, moving, as it were, from one morality and political economy to another in exchange for better infrastructure and higher incomes. The economic change played out in many developing cities where the private hospitals got stronger. At the same time, public and *vakıf* (philanthropic public trust) hospitals tried to make more progress and improve their infrastructure. Akdeniz University in Antalya, which was founded by Karpuzoğlu as a *public* university, began enjoying a growing rate of cadaveric transplants. Ege University, in İzmir in western Turkey, had similar success stories since it was able to integrate neoliberal ideas about transplant sourcing, together with a partial acceptance of brain death as the criterion of death that allowed the harvesting of organs, into rigid structures of public medical practice. Consequently, when the Ministry of Health wanted to establish a more "professional" database that would computerize and manage organ sharing across the whole country, physicians everywhere responded negatively. Akdeniz University opted out of the system, its surgeons arguing that they had had problems in basic matters such as tissue typing in organs they had received from Istanbul. But this was not the only problem: the organs had to travel great distances and Turkish airlines did not have many direct flights. Organs often had to be sent via Istanbul or Ankara to get to their final destinations nearby, increasing their time in transit.

The problem most responsible for low transplantation rates, however, was not an issue related to the management of databases or the efficiency of infrastructure, but to the diagnosis of brain death, physicians argued. There were not many brain-dead bodies to share. In transplant units at Ege and Akdeniz universities, physicians gradually achieved higher donation rates when they conducted workshops with the ICU and transplant physicians to train them on the proper definition and diagnosis of brain death. The unified database would jeopardize these efforts and decrease the number of cadaveric organs available in the southwestern part of the country.[46] Physicians wanted to keep and maintain the lists locally with a worldview they were familiar with, with physicians they could train, and a public they could relate to. They believed the success in the Aegean and Mediterranean regions was due to the open-mindedness of people there, which made it easier for physicians to speak of death to the public. The workshops gave physicians the courage and the "words" to achieve this. They were content with their local progress and did not want to receive or give away whatever they had invested in so far.

Other than finding local bodies for transplants, there was not much alternative but to travel abroad for transplants. Haberal was against outsourcing, that is, patients having transplants abroad. He had established his own database with a list of patients waiting for cadaveric transplants in his hospital. In some centers in Adana, Antalya, İzmir, and the east of the country he had strong ties, and so he could transform transplants into the realm of possibilities. Unlike Haberal, Eldegez at Istanbul University Medical School encouraged patients to go to other countries for transplants if they could afford it; he promised to take care of them at his unit during the post-transplant phase. This "intermediary" system, as he believed, was not a permanent solution, but the patient's life and health should be a physician's main priority.[47] That was why he encouraged patients, who would otherwise have to wait long years for a cadaveric transplant, to consider such an option. In some years the cadaveric transplant rate in Eldegez's unit dropped as low as 10 percent of annual transplant rates overall. Given these circumstances, many patients on the organ-sharing waiting lists in Ankara and Istanbul were urged to find donors on their own, to travel abroad, or introduce a "loved one" as a voluntary donor.[48]

To minimize monetary exchange in his unit, Eldegez had dedicated his work solely to transplants from brain-dead bodies, and outpatient and post-transplant care. His team believed that organ donation should be stimulated by every means to avoid potentially fatal unconventional infections after transplants from paid donors.[49] In this sense, if the patient bought an organ abroad, the early period of care was crucial for post-transplant survival; but more importantly, the main transplant donor pool should be from brain-dead bodies and not living ones. The more the transplant practice hewed to certain cultural sensibilities and taboos against the dead body, the more living bodies were used, including donors with hypertension, diabetes, or other renal diseases. This risked the health of the living body.[50]

Eldegez's socialist ideas were rooted in a morality that wanted to care for patients no matter where they had the operation, while also encouraging cadaveric transplants instead of living donors. Like many other physicians in Istanbul, he believed in strong public medical service instead of private ventures. The recent boom in private health-care services challenged the image of public services and attracted doctors and patients alike to private medicine. It even changed the patient profile, as Eldegez explained:

Most of our patients are poor. We have patients who come to us with money and they want to have a private operation. I send them to Russia, or they might go wherever they want to. We do not do such kind of business here. But of course in most living-related donation cases I have the feeling that they pay for the kidney, or, for example, the father is ill, then one of the sons gets an apartment from his brothers in exchange for his kidney. Or they promise to take care of him financially. Such internal deals are very common. This is actually against the organ transplantation law. However, we just do what we are required, we operate under the law Haberal made.

When Haberal had prepared the law to regulate organ harvesting from living or dead donors in 1979, he knew it would be difficult to procure cadaveric organs.[51] He believed that Turkish people, with their Muslim values, would think they were being betrayed by their own physicians if they tried to convince them to donate the organs of their loved ones. As the first transplant surgeon in Turkey he felt the weight of this responsibility and had borne these cultural and religious concerns in mind when he proposed the law on brain death. He had made the criteria for brain-death diagnosis more stringent than they were in the United States or any other country; this way the public would not accuse physicians of disrespecting tradition, the ancestors, and the dead. For Haberal, who linked himself to Atatürk's legacy in numerous ways,[52] it seemed more important to respect Turkish sensibilities than to improve the rate of cadaveric transplants. Living-related transplants were the best option and could maintain high survival rates and a running practice.

Overall, with transplantation the place of death in medicine had changed, moving from an undesirable condition to that of a commodity to be shared for the sake of the living. The new death bent the doctors' necks, made their eyelids heavy and their speech slow. It was the antithesis of the vocation of medicine, yet with transplantation it had become medicine's central preoccupation.

A young physician told me, "They [the medical establishment, transplant units] do not want to share the dead [ölüyü paylaşmak istemiyorlar]." He described the process:

When a brain-dead body is donated, the forms are filled out, and the coordination center is notified about the availability of the organs, includ-

ing the heart, liver, and kidneys. Doctors then do tissue typing. Matches
are found on the center's list of patients. Then the organs are distributed.
[Because the number of (brain-dead) donations are low, patients are encourage to go abroad for surgery.] Patients [also] find their way to India
through illegal channels . . . Dr. S., the reputed "organ mafia," was part of
our team. He was kicked out because he did illegal operations.

"Sharing the dead" (ölüyü paylaşmak), as it was often worded in speaking
about problems related to brain death, was a challenge. The young transplant surgeon in Istanbul, quoted above, had summarized the preoccupation well: this was an unresolved problem for all transplant centers. "Sharing the dead" had given rise to split biopolitics in an emerging economy of
the human flesh, from encouragement of legitimate living-related transplants to turning a blind eye to illegal operations, abroad or locally, under
the moral justification of saving lives.

Eldegez, unlike Haberal, was a proponent of transplantation based entirely on cadaveric donations: he opposed harvesting organs from living
bodies due both to risks to the donor and to ethical concerns about co-
ercion and informed consent. Haberal felt he had to practice transplants
but also be a role model physician who could coexist and respect beliefs
and culture. In other parts of the country, the dominant feelings toward
transplants were polarized at these two extremes, but there were many local efforts to improve conditions. Akdeniz University's success, like İzmir's,
was related to improvements in the diagnosis of brain death. Workshops
on brain death for the ICU and transplant physicians helped make progress. Ata Bozoklar, who had become the head of the coordination center in
İzmir, had initiated a double program to educate both physicians and the
public at once. Around the same time, Kalayoğlu had come back from the
United States to implement a transplant practice in a private hospital in
Istanbul. He and Bozoklar had begun a TV show on CNN-Türk to inform
the public along with these medical workshops. Through education and
"words," one could understand and speak of the new death, obtain more
brain-dead donors, and prevent many problems stemming from such institutional struggles as "sharing the dead" and the illicit organ market. The
ICU was at the heart of it.

Years ago, as he established his unit at Çapa, Eldegez had recognized
what a critical link the ICU was in his plans to conduct transplants from

cadaveric donors only: he expected the ICU doctors to inform him of all potential brain-dead donors in their care. But a study he conducted in 1991 revealed a resistant attitude toward the diagnosis of brain death in his own hospital. His transplant unit had been informed of only 10 percent of all cases of brain death. And of that 10 percent, only 1 percent had met the biological criteria for transplants and were usable. Why was he not informed? Why could he never establish good relations with the ICU physicians in his hospital? To an ICU physician, this was because of the conflict of interest between the two departments. The ICU physicians thought that the patient whose life had to be saved at all costs was seen as a medical object by the transplant teams. The latter wanted to diagnose brain death, the former tried to prevent it. The tension grew as both sides transformed brain death into an unclear, unattainable, *unknowable* form beyond the limits of medical language.

Brain Death

When physicians spoke of brain death, they used many different terms— *ölü* (the dead), *kadavra* (the cadaveric), *tıbbi ölüm hali* (medical death condition), or a more literal translation from the English, *beyin ölümü* (brain death). With all these they were referring to one and the same thing: the ambivalence of the brain death diagnosis. Though the criteria of brain death were "scientific" and universally acknowledged, it was difficult to translate them into a cultural context and give the condition a name that would correspond to a tangible and socially acceptable form of personhood.

Brain death is the criterion by which a body is declared dead and is made available for organ harvesting. It was first drafted in 1968 by a committee of experts at Harvard University in an effort to help increase the supply of viable organs for transplants. It was later adopted in many countries as the standard for harvesting organs such as the heart, liver, lungs, kidneys, and pancreas. In Turkey, the legal definition of brain death was inspired by the Harvard definition and modeled after international norms. Drafted in 1979 by Haberal, the Regulation on Organ Transplantations and Brain Death laid out the principles for organ and tissue harvesting from humans. The brain death diagnosis required confirmation of irreversible coma, absence of brainstem reflexes, and a positive apnea test in a normothermic, non-drugged patient, unanimously confirmed by the opinions of four specialists: a neurologist, a neurosurgeon, an anesthesiologist, and a cardiologist.[53] In the United States, by contrast, only one or two specialists were required, depending on state regulations. In addition, unlike in the United States and most European countries, Turkish doctors were not obliged by law to inform the hospital administration of all cases in which brain death seemed likely. The Turkish doctors understood that the requirements in their country made brain death diagnoses more difficult to make. The scientific and organizational requirements were giving physicians room to act according to their consciences. In this way, the requirements were reducing the chances of brain death diagnosis and keeping donor's relatives away from such a difficult decision. Consequently, it had become difficult to actually identify brain-dead bodies and perform transplants.

The reasons for the lack of brain-dead donors were complex. Physicians were reluctant to reduce death to brain functions and to speak of the dead body as if it were a person who was alive except for a single organ. Death could not be reduced to the lack of brain function as if a human were merely the sum total of his or her mind. There were fears, too, on the part of physicians, such as being accused of murder by a donor's family. "The dead," "the brain-dead body," "*kadavra*," "*donör*," "*hasta*" (patient), and "person" all mingled in the invention of the "*donör*" at the various institutional phases it passed through. Like ICU physicians, family members were confused when they had to sign the papers authorizing the removal of life support. Did the papers mean that a patient's relatives were consenting to his or her death? If the doctors needed a consent form to let the patient die, didn't this mean he or she was still alive? The patient's relatives could not understand this legal-medical maneuver, and many physicians could not explain it. This issue caused many physicians to feel conflicted about the truth behind brain death—the truth behind a scientific fact. Besides this legal obligation of family consent to withdraw life support, which would not be required in natural death, physicians confused it with the vegetative state, a reversible coma from which many had observed patients waking. They could not explain to their patients this concept of brain death, which contradicted their own experiences.

In time, public fears mingled with the competing interests of ICU doctors and transplant surgeons. Already in 1982 the term used to describe brain death had been changed from *beyin ölümü* (literally, brain death) to *tıbbi ölüm hali* (medical death condition) in the hope of emphasizing brain death as "real" death and not "the death of the brain." In the new translation, the word *ölüm* (death) was absorbed by the power of the word *tıbbi* (medical) and its hegemonic, technical, and institutional connotations. This semantic change, however, did not work; the diagnosis criteria did not become more flexible,[54] nor did the number of brain-dead donors improve.

Many physicians were uneasy with these translations and had a hard time speaking to me about them. As the head of the transplant coordination team of the Ege Region, Bozoklar trained physicians on brain death. Trainees typically understood the scientific basis for brain death, but they had a hard time dealing with its metaphysics. The reduction of life to a biological function in the brain brought them uncomfortably close to the idea of extinction, which was a difficult thing to comprehend. It was normal for trainees to have issues with this kind of definition of death when they could observe the patient still breathing (even though the patient's breathing was maintained via a respirator); they were confused and concerned. Kalayoğlu, too, encountered similar confusion. He could not forget, for example, a recent encounter with a senior transplant physician who had implied that he did not understand "brain death" and wanted Kalayoğlu to tell him the true story behind it.

The brain/self analogy of clinical brain death contradicted the body/*jann* relationship. *Jann* was everywhere in the body and partly it also constituted the essence of the self. With the change in wording to the "death of the brain," it became a "medical condition." The new words decentralized death and shifted the center of the diagnosis from the brain to the entire body. In the end, *jann* was not located in one organ but throughout the body: it was in the lungs, the heart, the pulse, and also, as Bozoklar told me, in the *nefes* (the breath). Brain death reduced death to the lack of brain function and not to the passage of *jann* out of the body. For this reason, Bozoklar preferred to describe brain death as *"son nefesini verdi"* (the patient gave away his last breath), which meant that the *jann* had left the body and there was no longer life in it. He avoided the terms "brain death" and "medical death condition."

There were other more intuitive limits. A patient connected to the respirator would be referred to as the *vakaa* (case) rather than the *hasta* (patient). If physicians verified any of the brain death indications, then the patient would be called a *donör adayı* (donor candidate), the word *donör* borrowed directly from English. If the family had given consent, the patient would become a *donör*. Physicians in the ICU would never call a brain-dead person attached to a respirator by any other term than *donör*, a doctor at the Istanbul University Reanimation Center told me. According to Bozoklar, the literal translation of the word donor, *verici*, would be a very difficult word to use. It entailed exchange, profit, materiality. Like *hasta* (patient), *verici* (donor) did not fit into the scheme: both terms were affect-laden. These words suggested a condition in which the dead person would be detached from the *unknowable* divine realm and enter the domain of common sense where all sorts of things, among them exchange, took place. Even though everyone spoke of brain death as death itself, this rhetorical process was only made possible by transforming the Turkish word *verici* into an English adaptation, *donör*. This way the brain-dead body could become a cadaver, a Western medical object with a Latin name to be used for biomedical progress. Likewise the brain-dead donor was commonly referred to as the *kadavra* (cadaveric donor), a word that was semantically and thus genealogically linked to anatomy's research object, the *kadavra* (cadaver).

Yet, this borrowed science was not without problems even in the United States. In English, there is a fine distinction maintained between the terms "cadaver" and "the cadaveric organ": the adjectival form acknowledged the technical need to keep the organ viable, perfused with blood while the donor's body was still cadaver-like. One could also provoke arguments among American physicians over the precision of declaring brain death. Organ allocation physicians and administrators were adamant that indeterminacy should not be admitted lest the delicate permissible procedures be called into question. Turkish doctors used the term *kadavra* as a sign of their discomfort with the fine distinction and as an indication that the "medical death condition" may actually be an unreliable form of death. Even in English, the term "cadaver" was used instead of the word "corpse," again a fine affective distinction.

The dead body on a respirator with its heart beating and skin warm could not be diagnosed with brain death. The translations from the English fell into the void; the brain-dead donor could not materialize. The main misunderstanding, physicians commonly agreed, was caused by the term "brain death" itself and not by any physical observation that made the physicians suspicious of the science behind it. But still, physicians believed that by inventing the right vocabulary they could actually materialize the condition since this was how science had been internalized traditionally. In the Turkish experience, the object materialized ontologically within the culture of medicine first in a plausible translation. This way it could be made a part of the biomedical practice—it could be made local. In the case of brain death, this term signified to such an affect-laden object, the brain-dead donor, that it was impossible to live with. For the body to become a viable source of organs, a commodity and a *knowable* thing, it had to become an object of science. This could happen through the borrowed nature of scientific concepts and objects from the West. Then detached from its original imaginaries and by means of language, it could be made a part of the symbolic. This way the object would acquire a name. Physicians were trying to invent the object by means of a name that originated in a scientific and bureaucratic context far away, culturally, theologically, and linguistically. Scientific terminology was aided by legal maneuvers to materialize the brain-dead donor as a medical object, but the legal change did not help support the decontextualization of the patient into a donor—who no longer should be seen a person but an object. Efforts to invent metaphors to describe brain death did not clarify the confusion caused by the paperwork required for consent.

In this emerging field's ideals, the medical passage of the brain-dead body from the *unknowable* domain of death to the *knowable* world of the cadaver would have been an *aufklärung*, the German term also used for the Enlightenment, the slogan of modernization both in Europe and in the Turkish republic. This passage would have allowed the reincorporation of the deceased back into social life through techniques that regulated emotions and human affairs. Then, with the naming of brain death the dead body and its *jann* would emerge from the realm of the *unknowable* divine and move into the *unknown* domain of medical practices to take its place next to anatomy and forensic medicine as it has throughout the history of modernity in Turkey.

The complexity involving brain death diagnosis was, in a way, keeping things as they used to be: the dead body in the *unknowable* world of the divine; medical objects within the world of lively exchange. "Brain death" would have transformed the person into an emptied object that had taken its last breath in bureaucracy and in religious orthodoxy, and thus the body could be viable for organ harvesting in the short span of time between death and burial. For this reason, its invention was partly grounded in religious orthodoxy and partly in people's ideas of death and the afterlife. The deep theological grounds of Islamic law performed a pragmatic role for this "life-saving" practice of the biopolis for physicians and patients alike.

The Theological Limits of Life and Death

The brain-dead donor in its "wholeness" and "liveliness" existed in a liminal realm hard to naturalize as a medical object in Turkey, even for a brief time. This was partly due to the place the body occupied in Islamic theology—an *emanet* (a borrowed thing from God) animated by the *jann*. Being an *emanet* in life, in death the body had exited this worldly profane realm to be returned to its owner in the divine universe. Transplants had to pass through these stable moral worlds upon which religious orthodoxy had been producing personal meanings of life and death for centuries. People gave meaning to their lives through these separations as nature and theology revealed. Brain death fell into a place between the two worlds and undid many categories for this reason.

In Turkish Islamic tradition, as elsewhere, the Qur'an, the *hadith*, and the Sunnah are the main sources of the moral and legal principles for the daily lives of Muslims, although customary and state law have also always been recognized in the *shar'ia*.[55] These texts defined personhood on theological grounds. When a person died, for instance, it was forbidden to violate the corpse or the grave intentionally, as in all other religions. But the line that divided the doctrine from pragmatism was thin, so a practice like autopsy that helped reveal truth by solving a crime and exposing the criminal was no longer regarded as violation in modern times.[56]

Traditionally, the Turkish ulema did not interfere in medical decision making. In the Islamic world, from Ibn-Khaldun (1332–1406) on, scholars have debated whether medical matters lay in the realm of reason or of religion, and the general conclusion has been that *vahiy* (revelations) and *şeriat* (*shar'ia*, Islamic law) were not useful bases for judging the practice of medicine.[57] It was not the ulema's delegated power to decide whether a person was dead; that remained in the purview of medicine. In 1980 when the Diyanet (the government's Presidency of Religious Affairs) approved organ harvesting and transplantation of organs from living and dead bodies, they were more concerned about protecting the bodily integrity of the *person*, alive or dead, than questioning the technical and theological validity of brain death.[58] The Diyanet left the diagnosis of brain death in the hands of doctors, trusting their consciences (*vicdan*) and expertise. Faced with an imperative (*zaruret*) such as saving a life, one could perform a transplant from a brain-dead or living donor as long as it did not violate the donor's rights.

In the 1970s, Abdülkerim Zeydan, a scholar of Islamic studies at the University of Baghdad, had argued that in the case of imminent starvation, Islam permitted the eating of human flesh.[59] The justifying motive for cadaveric donation was interpreted as the same as that for cannibalism: by eating human flesh one would be saved from dying, and by receiving an organ from a dead person one would heal. It was essential, however, that the harvesting of the organs did not violate bodily dignity, that all medical criteria were met, and that there was no material exchange involved.[60] While the rest of the Muslim world continued to debate brain death and cadaveric organ harvesting, Turkish scholars of Islam decided to adopt an existing international *fatwa* that covered these issues.[61] Later on, at a meeting in Oman in 1986, the Pan-Islamic Council of Jurisprudence moved to leave the diagnosis of brain death to medical experts,[62] and in Mecca in 1988 the same council issued guidelines defining conditions for organ harvesting.[63] This *fatwa* forbade the commodification of organs from living bodies: the sale of organs was illegal, and human life could not be bought and sold.[64] Only organs that could be removed without risking the donor's life could be used for living-related transplants.[65] Any excessive risk would violate the basic principle of the right to life and bodily integrity.

While this was the general approach to issues such as autopsy and transplantation in Turkey, the Ministry of Justice in Saudi Arabia, to which the Turkish ulemas sometimes turned for guidance, had declared a very different view on the use of cadavers for medical research. It allowed a corpse to be used for solving a crime or learning about an infectious disease. In regard to anatomy, however, it concluded that despite Islam's respect for progress in science and education, anatomical dissection should be limited to the bodies of executed criminals. The reason, it argued, was that dissection devalued the respectability of the body. Those who were sentenced to the death penalty were regarded as non-persons outside the moral and economic value system. In this world, these stigmatized bodies were somehow inferior to others, which made these particular bodies a potential source for organ harvesting. From a theological perspective, the dead body was at least as valuable as the living body. Muhammad told in one of his *hadith* that breaking a dead man's bone was like breaking his bone when he was alive. Yet this equal value of the body in life and in death did not hold for people who had violated the norms of righteousness and thereby abandoned the protection offered by conformity to norms.

The consent of religious authorities was drawn upon categories of personhood and the imperative to save a human life. Despite its theologically grounded and human-centered roots, it did not have a positive influence in encouraging physicians to make brain death diagnoses, except for cases of suicide, nor did it encourage people to donate their bodies for organ transplants. Nevertheless, physicians always supported their arguments with the religious consent in favor of transplants.

Despite religious orthodoxy's permission for the brain death diagnosis and for transplantation in general, there was a side of culture, a side of people themselves, where conscience and fears prevented them from organ donation. This side of the self emerged in myths and legends, especially on death and the dead body. To me, myths, legends, and stories were a deeper side of culture carved into individual lives. To have a glimpse of these stories and their invention in the high-tech world, I began looking into different sites where I could find out more about the effect of the dead body upon medical practices. Many physicians were concerned about the commodification of the human body for medical ends, seeing it as a violation, yet they also wanted to practice medicine and establish high-tech practices. Urban legends and scandals emerged from these fears, acting as a brake to slow down the construction of the transplant practice and weaving the trails patients had to take toward their new lives. They regulated life, setting its limits by inflicting fears about violating and being violated at once. Transplants, in this sense, overlapped with other spheres of medicine that utilized the human body and its parts for medical ends, that had to transform subjects into objects. I was especially intrigued by stories I had been told that extended into the harvesting of human bones for orthopedic surgery. There, a whole economy was construed upon fears of violating the dead body despite the scientific and religious reasoning and authority.

Myth and the Limits of Culture

Many fears surrounded the harvesting, safekeeping, and use of human bones. These fears were rooted in belief in the afterlife, the pollution resulting from the mixing of body parts of the living and the dead, and the violation of the rights of dead people. While transplant physicians have been occupied with words, and with translations of brain death into Turkish in order to materialize the local brain-dead donor for transplants, orthopedic surgeons who used imported allografts were justifying the legitimacy of their vocation through myths. With stories that would transform their outlook toward harvesting bones from dead bodies, people in this field were utilizing scandals and transforming them into myths. This way they could keep the "easy market" in allografts a running business without interfering with taboos surrounding the dead body. Yet, to keep this "easy market" alive and functioning, they would also have to discourage local science and physicians from harvesting bones from local bodies.

A surgeon who also traded in allografts told me of a recent encounter with an American businessman who sold allografts to the Turkish. His company was interested in expansion and asked the surgeon's opinion whether Turkey would be a good place to start a tissue bank in the region: "Once, last year, as the American salesman was here for a meeting, he asked me if we would be interested in building a factory in Turkey. . . . I mean a factory for human bones, a factory that is supposed to turn bones harvested from us, Turks, into material for export and local consumption. A factory! . . . I told him, it is not possible in Turkey, not in our culture. I told him, if it were possible, we would have done it ourselves. . . . And moreover not a factory! So, we will have to import these bones no matter what."

In Turkey, bones were hardly harvested for implants to be stored in tissue banks. The implant field had been growing at a different speed and history from that of internal organs worldwide. It was a sector that originated in metal implants and then shifted toward parts harvested from animals. Recently with the progress in regenerative technologies, human bones were being used as commercial products as well. I had encountered more wild stories on this practice than on any other field of medicine. This subtle difference was born on fears of violating the dead. Its legendary stories had in time acquired mythic powers regarding death, and had began affecting its economy.

The impetus for allowing the import of allografts arose from an incident in the early 1990s at Hacettepe University Hospital in Ankara. A body was donated for organ transplantation. The harvesting teams for the heart, liver, pancreas, kidneys, and cornea lined up and harvested their respective organs. An orthopedist was in the operating room chatting with them. The vital organ teams suggested that since the body had been donated, they might as well harvest its bones. The orthopedist liked the idea, spoke with his team, and after all the others were done harvesting, they went in for the femurs and tibias (the upper and lower leg bones). When they finished, they sewed the legs back up to prepare the body for delivery to the mosque where two family members would wash it and wrap in a shroud. However, as the doctors attempted to lift the body, the legs hung limply, and they realized it would be impossible to carry it anywhere. They had to find a solution right away, and one member of the team suggested they implant the handle from a broom in the operating room. They cut the broomstick to the appropriate lengths, cut the leg muscles open again, and inserted the pieces so that the muscles would be supported.

The cadaver was delivered to the mosque, and the deceased's family members began the traditional cleansing ritual. While they were washing the body, however, the strangest thing happened: the sticks cut through the muscle tissue and broke through the skin. The family members were horrified: pieces of wood were sticking out of their loved one's damaged flesh. They ran to the imam and told him what had happened, and the imam alerted the hospital administration. Before long the whole orthopedist community had heard the story and it was quickly covered up. Nevertheless, it became a legend that I heard about from doctors each time I asked them why bones could not be harvested from cadavers in Turkey. That incident was both the beginning and the end of the practice.

This story mythologized the pretext that regulated the Turkish allograft market. Unlike the harvesting of other organs, the removal of bones provoked a feeling that violence had been done to the body and that the immortality of the body and the integrity of one's kin had been disrespected. As one physician said,

> When you harvest a kidney or a liver, you close the body and no one sees what has happened to it. But when you harvest bones, the wholeness of the body is destroyed. The family [of the deceased person] realizes that. It is unacceptable. They see it when they wash the body. You can put cheap material inside the body after harvesting the bones. But all this requires investment in Turkey, which is the main problem.

What the patient's family asks is whether the body will be in one piece after harvesting. . . . If you say I will take the legs, it is not okay. . . . When you lose the bones, there would be no problem for the anatomy labs to use the rest of the body for dissection as well. . . . But it does not work that way. . . . Only the corneas are available because there is no visible loss. . . . For that, no one asks the permission of family members. . . . It is done right away. . . . No one sees the cadaver's eyes, because they are closed. . . . Then come the internal organs. . . . Since the doctors sew up the body, no one sees the inside of the body after harvesting. . . . But patients' relatives would refuse if the legs were missing. . . . When you look from outside, the body has to look normal.

It was essential to respect rituals and preserve the wholeness of the body for the washing ritual in the mosque. By washing, cleaning, and then wrapping the body in a clean white shroud, family members would be paying their last respects to the deceased before the funeral. They would be preparing the corpse for the afterlife. In the end, even if the dead body lacked *jann*, it was still full of memories that had to be preserved so that the human would remain human. Over the years, the story at Hacettepe had exceeded legendary qualities and become a postmodern myth but also a pretext that regulated the imported allograft market. With similar stories, the Turkish orthopedists were telling me of their concern about the local usage of human subjects for medical ends, and why it would be better simply to import these products. An orthopedist from Ankara expressed his concerns:

Sometimes companies come up with ideas. . . . The tissue bank we work with suggested having a factory in Turkey. . . . And we told them about our problem. . . . The technology is simple, but if you cannot find a donor there is no way. . . . We could even market the bones abroad. I think they will choose Italy [to build the factory]. . . . There is infrastructure there. Another offer was from Germany; they said, "You find us the donors and we will take the bones, screen them, and bring them back." This is also illegal. . . . We cannot trust them and . . . it is illegal. . . . Our laws are hard to change.

Besides fears against violating the wholeness of the body, physicians were concerned about the domestic infrastructure that had to meet the scientific criteria required to establish and maintain a tissue bank. Surgeons and merchants involved in the business of allografts had not known of the scientific practice in tissue engineering in Turkey. Already in the 1990s, as the market in grafts shifted to allografts, Turkish scientists had noticed the growing demand for human tissue for surgery, and a group of them decided to launch a multi-year project to implement a tissue bank that could produce allografts for the domestic market. But somehow their efforts were blocked by the government, which seemed to be interested in the importation of allografts instead of the production of local ones. In 1997, the International Atomic Energy Agency (IAEA) provided the Çekmece Nuclear Training and Research Center (CNAEM) with the equipment necessary for tissue processing. The IAEA sent experts to train Turkish scientists on tissue banking and tissue-processing methods. The agency had already been assisting Turkey in the introduction of radiation technology for sterilizing disposable medical products. The tissue engineering efforts built on this relationship. The efforts that began in 1997 were successful. But scientists had a hard time getting permission from the Ministry of Health to distribute these locally produced allografts. Turkey was spending hundreds of thousands of U.S. dollars for this purpose while continuing to import radiation-sterilized tissue grafts from other countries.[66] The disagreement between the government and the Scientific and Technological Research Council of Turkey (TÜBİTAK), which is the agency for managing, funding, and conducting research in Turkey, was part of the problem. The government was slow to encourage local scientific projects; instead, it encouraged multinationals to enter the local market and sell their high-tech products. The council, in contrast, wanted to forge ahead with local science and engineering efforts despite its very limited budget. Medium-sized importers and small businesses were seen as essential for Turkish health care despite corruption and abuse.

While the difficulties of "sharing the dead" *locally* had initiated the utilization of living-related transplants to prevent conflicts of interest in hospital corridors, the "absence of life"—the absence of proteins—in *imported* products had made the allografting business easy and profitable, but also relatively unregulated and more easily abused. To get demineralized bones, leg bones were harvested and then demineralized by radiation, screened for viruses, and preserved at -80 degrees Celsius in large deep-freezes. Frozen, freeze-dried, or demineralized, these bones had no life in them—they were just an inert matrix. In the body, after implantation, living tissue would grow over the matrix, giving life to it. This was different from a kidney, a thing that almost had a life of its own. While trafficking vital organs was strictly forbidden, the trade of these inert body parts was legal and loosely regulated.

In 2000, the Ministry of Health categorized imported bones as "healing medical material" (*iyileştirici tıbbi malzeme*), a category with its own set of guidelines different from those for blood products or pharmaceuticals. Human bones used for orthopedic purposes were called "human-originating healing medical material" (*insan menşekli iyileştirici tıbbi malzeme*), a label that, to the uninitiated, did not make the fact of bone harvesting explicit. Like the wording of *donör* instead of *verici* or *kadavra* instead of *beyin ölümü*, there were efforts to translate these products into Turkish or invent new names to internalize them. While the language of the trading protocols was much more matter-of-fact, most orthopedists were annoyed when the word *kemik* (bone) was used instead of the English word "graft" to refer to these "human-originating healing materials." Besides, traditionally orthopedic surgeons would not speak to the patients about the origin of these bones anyway, I had been told. They were simply referred to as *graft* (as in English) without indicating the source of the implant (metal, animal, or human).

Unlike other pharmaceutical and blood products, for years graft materials were not tested or controlled at customs. In 1999, a company that imported from the United States requested that the Ministry of Health regulate these materials more stringently. There was an urgent need for regulation as new competitors from places like Hungary and Bulgaria were entering the graft market.[67] Eastern European prices were low; the bone graft materials being imported into Turkey were not being tested, and it was impossible to know whether a virus might be transmitted in the implant. The only complication orthopedists would detect after an operation was an infection, and it was hard to determine its real cause.[68]

There was much hype involving the allograft market. Since it was *possible* to import these "lifeless" products, they were imported. Local science was undermined by accusations of a lack of infrastructure to pursue such high-tech research, and by a risk to public health. These "emptied" "imported" body parts were now merely products in plastic bags, alienated from any origins and past. In this biopolis, stories on missing legs could easily assume mythic characteristics and be told to historicize the emergence, the creation, of a market economy that had to commodify human life to prevent the violation of the dead body at home in Turkey.

THE ECONOMY OF HUMAN FLESH AND BONES

From the 1980s onward, Turkey had begun to be a land of possibilities for private investors and industry. Turkish businessmen were encouraged by tax exemptions to invest in all kinds of ventures. Within a decade, many hospitals had been founded in the spirit of Özal's neoliberal policies; and by the year 2000, more than 100 of the 137 licensed hospitals in Istanbul were private. Along with the spread of private clinics and health-care services, private insurance companies entered the market too. At that time, the 26 public, social security, and university hospitals in Istanbul began to provide care only for those who could not afford any private insurance. Most of their patients were public servants, workers, farmers, and people who worked for medium- or small-sized employers. One doctor who had just left a state hospital in Ankara and moved to Istanbul in the late 1990s to work in a private clinic told me the following:

> Private practice is a good source of income, but the main money in medicine goes to hospital owners. Most of the public insurance and all of the private insurance covers the treatments. The price range of these operations has been controlled by the Turkish Medical Association since 1998, because the private insurance companies found out that many doctors were writing false prescriptions for patients; things like declaring that an operation was for a traffic accident victim when it actually was a cosmetic nose surgery became normal. Fraud had become a part of the routine in the medical community and the Ministry of Health could not control it. So private insurance companies have actually forced the Turkish Medical Association to set up a price range in U.S. dollars to control fraud because they could not make profits any longer. One could imagine that the increasing number of private hospitals would be an even better damper for the fraud, but it happened just the opposite way. The private hospital owners have turned medicine into a business and they do not want to share with doctors; nor do they want to be accused of fraud by the insurance companies. So as they become stronger, they are changing the rules of the game.

The health-care industry was manipulated and abused yet it grew with the emergence of big patrons and medium-sized importers and clinics. From 1997 to 2003 health-care services expenditures in Turkey increased multiple times.[69] By 2004, health-care product imports *excluding pharmaceuticals* were valued at U.S.$805 million.[70] This rapid increase was due to the growth of the private health-care industry from small-scale importers to hospital ownership.

With the increase in the number of private health-care providers, physicians began moving toward the "better" infrastructure. As a result physicians' status as caregivers changed. But not all physicians were interested in the private sector; the movement from public service to the private was influenced by the degree of control and authority to which they were willing to submit. In private hospitals, management exerted significant control over the decisions physicians used to make in their own units and according to their own consciences. The "idealistic" transplant surgeons, who used to practice transplant medicine as a public service and for no personal benefit, began moving away from these posts for better wages and better infrastructure, eventually becoming a part of the private venture movement while bringing public medicine's elite and paternalistic attitude with them into the elegant and luxurious private hospital units.

The transition from public to private authority provoked debate about whether the state and its physicians had more authority over medicine than patrons of private health care. It was a hegemonic fight more than anything else. The age-old authority enjoyed by physicians, who wielded it as a natural aspect of the social contract between themselves and the public, was being questioned and rapidly transformed by the rise of private domains. The country's social mosaic was changing with its biomedical and technological reconstruction. The changes that became so pronounced in the 1990s and early 2000s actually began several years earlier with the reforms instituted by Özal, who was a great admirer of American technological progress.[71] His economic reforms of the 1980s began transforming Turkish political and economic life away from the centralized state authority that had been governed by the Kemalist political elite. He relied on private industry overall and invested state resources in development; he encouraged exports and remained conservative in imports. As in the case of allografts, imports had been the traditional way of acquiring manufactured technological goods from abroad. The trust in imported products stemmed in this faith in Western technology.[72] Özal, in contrast, wanted industry's and tourism's mobility to transform Turkey's economy.

At the same time, many *vakıf*, or nongovernmental foundations, were established in the education and health-care sectors. Both Başkent University and Akdeniz University were launched during this period. *Vakıf* were encouraged because of the way they were seen as bridging institutions: launched by private individuals, run as nonprofits, and supported by tax exemptions of the state. Haberal, whose name circulated in Turkey's presidential elections of 2000, directed Başkent University's funds. Most of the medical appliances and dialysis fluids used at Başkent were produced in Haberal's own factories and sold to his own hospital. The consumption of his own goods was thus a source of income. But because the university and its hospital were ostensibly charitable organizations, he also profited from state subventions. When I visited Haberal, his office was decorated with the medals and certificates of honor he had received from many Turkish business societies. He was named businessman of the year by the Turkish Industrialists' and Businessmen's Association (TÜSİAD), the most prestigious business award in Turkey. The move from the public Hacettepe Medical School to the *vakıf* Başkent University had allowed Haberal a great freedom to expand his transplant and dialysis units. He had transformed his practice into a nationwide center for transplants this way.

Historically, *vakıf* dated all the way back to the time of the Ottoman rule. But in 1989 the Berlin Wall came down, and afterward borders changed, effecting mobility and capital flow. *Vakıf*'s nonprofit structure became an ideal platform upon which the liberal market economy could flourish. While the flow of market capital into social development transformed centralized governance and allowed participation, it excluded plurality, widened the gap between the rich and the poor, and segregated people in physical space. A new generation of the wealthy began actively challenging the state's status quo, the military authorities, and the Kemalist intellectual elites; among the challengers were a middle class with conservative Muslim values, nationalists partly supported by the extreme right and the "underground," and diverse investors from abroad.

The name of the change was liberalism, professionalism, privatization. This time people traveled across continents and vocations to return to a place they had left, a place where they could start new ventures yet in a different synthesis. In this way, the biopolis, the universe in which transplantation operated, had moved from vision to practice and materialized through mobility, neoliberal economies, and globalization. Neoliberal markets in particular moved through spheres of social life to undo the past. The idea of business and business management lied at the heart of this movement. Hospital managers had become at least as important as physicians in this biopolis.

Ali was one of the first professional hospital managers in Turkey. When we met in 2000 he had just returned from the United States, where he learned hospital management at Columbia University. He had come back to Turkey to take a job helping to establish a new private hospital in Istanbul. Given the growth in private medicine in the late 1990s, the job offer was worth moving back to Turkey for. He was recruiting most of his medical staff from the new community of repatriated Turkish doctors, who, like him, had returned to Turkey in those years.

Ali thought Turkish physicians were unfamiliar with professional hospital management in the way it was practiced in the United States. Traditionally in Turkey, reputable medical practice was established in public hospitals. Their management was influenced by the political environment as it changed after every national election. Actually, the significant change in hospital ownership in Turkey had dated back to the early 1970s, when a physician started buying up small hospitals, establishing a large chain by the 1990s. By 2000, the same physician owned more than fifty medical institutions in Turkey, around twenty of them in Istanbul. Dr. S., the so-called organ mafia doctor, operated in this chain of hospitals until he opened his own clinic. Private hospitals, in this sense, were also spaces that embraced what was excluded by public hospitals; they were ready to offer "more" than the usual practice of health care.

Private hospital ownership was profitable. A private hospital received part of the surgeon's fee for each operation performed there. The hospital charged patients for accommodation expenses and got a share of the coverage from the patients' insurance companies; in the end, the hospital had three sources of income from each operation. Transplantation was an especially attractive practice, not least because of its prestigious reputation. It was the proof of skilled teams, devoted physicians, and well-equipped hospitals. For this reason, management was interested in establishing transplant units as soon as transplant units were allowed by law to have them. The new and unknown hospital would prove quality health services this way. "Organ transplantation is not conducted in private hospitals yet, and state insurance covers all transplantation operation costs, but we will try to change this," he said in 2000, excited about the pressures the private sector could exert to challenge public health care. According to Ali,

> What we want is to be able to open private organ and tissue banks and do organ transplantation in private hospitals like ours. . . . There are illegal operations in Turkey because of the gap between the poor and the rich. The wealthy will pay for it by whatever means they can. . . . So why does the state still insist on such centralized regulations? When we make it private, we will be able to control the legal status of the operations at least. There will be no criminal activity. . . . They put an end to Dr. S.'s medical career. It is most unfortunate. He is the best transplant surgeon in this country, and of course he will do transplantation. . . . This is his job.

Dr. S. was neither a hero nor a villain in Ali's world. The picture he drew illustrated the emergence of a biomedical imaginary with skilled management, strong ownership, and physicians ready to cross over moral zones of common sense for a "vocation." This vision contradicted the legislation of the early 2000s that banned transplantation in private hospitals.

In this emerging world the exchange value of the body was changing, partly due to new gift exchange demands within families strapped for money, and partly due to the entry of multinational pharmaceutical and medical organizations, which disseminated a market economy in things that previously could not be sold or transferred. A group of influential medical practitioners backed by sizeable capital could be a powerful force for furthering the change toward transplants in private hospitals. Ali even envisioned the eventual completely legal marketing of human organs.

By 2003, the world of medicine had changed so much and so rapidly that Ali's visions were already materializing: under the pressure of the growing health-care market, private hospitals were permitted to have transplant units. A successful unit required a large and well-trained staff of the sort typically found at public hospitals only. These well-to-do hospitals were paying around three times the public-sector salary of a transplant surgeon to draw physicians away. Memorial Hospital's new liver transplant unit was the nation's largest and most skilled. Its staff included Kalayoğlu, who had founded and directed the liver transplant unit at the University of Wisconsin, Madison, and Acarlı, the former head of the liver team at Istanbul University Medical School. Another recently founded *vakıf* hospital, Anadolu Sağlık Merkezi-Johns Hopkins planned on establishing its own kidney transplant unit with an American-trained team. Yaman Tokat's team at Florence Nightingale Hospital in Istanbul was another success story of transplant practices which also marked the move from public to private hospitals.

While the private hospitals moved on with their own political agendas to establish transplant units, private investors' desire to make a profitable business of body parts began to raise complex sets of issues. Public hospitals and their transplant units expressed low confidence in the future of transplants in private hospitals. Turkey was in a socioeconomic transition, and transplantation was seen as its idealistic, almost utopian face in scientific practice with analogies drawn to space research. It signified something beyond mere surgery and medical technology. Transplantation as a medical practice had proven what could be done despite poverty and cultural taboos surrounding death; it showed how science and technology could mold the social body for the well-being of the social life; it showed how *jann* could be utilized to implement technologies of the self. Social life was collective and so were transplants. They were a public domain and could only be controlled by the mechanisms that regulated matters of life and death. Taking the "public" body into the "private" domain for organ harvesting or transplantation was leaving this social and cultural practice in the hands of capital owners—it was a dangerous moral zone. The private domain could impose its normative spiritual morality over the public domain, while changing the social mosaics of matters of death that had been kept almost sacred to remind people of who they were. It was where the heart of culture beat. If one transformed this sphere, one would no longer be in a moral zone of debate on bioethical matters—an ethical plateau[73]—but one would be overruling a whole worldview and further advantaging the wealthy.

The lack of cadaver organs for transplants, difficulties with brain death diagnosis, and the presence of a large and accessible illicit kidney market in Turkey raised other questions as well, related to how much of a share private hospitals should have in the newly unified national organ-sharing database. With privatized transplantation, wealthy patients would be able to pay the hospital and the chief surgeon in order to be placed at the top of the waiting list in a hospital with few transplant patients, increasing their chances of getting a cadaveric kidney within the system of organ allocation. Transplant surgeons in public hospitals were opposed to giving private hospitals the access to the newly established nationwide database for this reason.

Transplant medicine arose in Turkey in the initial years of the complex socioeconomic environment of the 1980s. Everyone engaged in law, politics, education, and health care contributed to its biomedical imaginary as it unfolded to become a solid practice. Patients I had known had encountered different slices of this economic growth as their personal lives overlapped certain physicians, hospitals, and public health policies. Some patients got listed in the collective database for a cadaveric organ, some traveled long distances for private health care, some could only hope for a brain-dead donor, and some were in the market to buy a kidney. The complex epistemics of transplant political economy and its language were shaping the way patients gave meaning to their experiences. These determined where, when, and how they would become a transplant patient, and how they learned to speak of their transformed new selves. New relational objects that were introduced to patients' inner lives were in a rather obvious way changing them into an entity in a large population, into a machine-dependent body, a subject of the state, yet a subject still under the influence of older traditions. They were living through images of media scandals and of political struggles over transplantation, which exposed to them the unfinished institutional features of their own inner universe. Transplant patients had to come to terms with and internalize a variety of biomedical objects: donations, sacrificial gestures, and the ambiguities of a *kadavra* as well as other objects from the dialysis machine to organs as quasi-commodities. Their lives had been restored through these objects. In this biopolis, physicians' central and most challenging occupation was death: a thing that should not be traded, trafficked, misunderstood, or exchanged; a thing that should be left among the objects of the *unknowable* realm; a thing that should be kept safe to remind people what life was about. Most physicians claimed to be more concerned with the violation of respect toward the dead than with the commodification of the living body. Patients survived renal failure only through negotiating such biopolitical conundrums.

Because of these conundrums, in the thirty-year history of transplants, the overwhelming majority of organ harvesting was from living related donors. Many of these were selling their organs, a trade widely practiced in Turkey and in other places in the Middle East even without the involvement of dealers, merchants, or businessmen. It was acknowledged that a renal patient could locate a person who might be willing to "donate" a kidney in exchange for some sort of material compensation. This could be a family member, a distant relative, or someone from the patient's village. A patient with sufficient money could find a donor, introduce him or her to the transplant physicians as an unrelated living donor, the third-degree kinship tie, and have the donor sign the required voluntary consent papers. To Eldegez, the ban on organ selling contradicted the surgeon's oath to preserve a patient's life, constructing an untenable definition of ethical behavior: surgeons who performed transplants from living donors could not avoid being complicit in these illegal pacts between patients and donors. Moreover, knowledge of a donor's or a patient's personal life, or becoming intimate with their problems, could influence a doctor's conscience and even his own sense of agency. This was the reason why Eldegez's unit was dedicated to operating only with cadaveric organs. Besides the internal deals between the recipient and the donor, there were special exceptional cases such as that of caring for patients who had received illegal transplants elsewhere. Physicians believed the system of transplant medicine was inadequate, yet they could not agree on how best to adapt it to the Turkish culture.

While Eldegez was concerned about post-transplant care and donor health, Haberal was mainly concerned about the misgivings of the public about the system and the lack of communication among physicians and patients resulting in organizational problems. The ban on organ and tissue sale was strict. Yet it was difficult for physicians to know the true nature of the relationship between a donor and a recipient. If the selling of body parts were legalized, people would start killing each other for organs, he thought. With this possibility out of the question and with the prevailing lack of brain-dead donors, the number of transplants from living donors increased day by day, Haberal believed. He told me,

The trade exists in Russia, England, and India. Such activities happen in those countries. It also occurs in Romania, Moldavia, and Israel. We do not have it here in Turkey. Our law is important. We value the law.

On the other hand, Dr. S. is an unfortunate case. I have known him for ten years. He came to me. He asked me to help him. I gave him a respirator for the Kartal ssk Hospital where he was establishing the transplant unit. After rumors spread about him, I wanted to meet him [in person]. I warned him about the law and the way doctors work in Turkey. He did not listen to me. So I stopped talking to him. . . . He became a businessman. He is not in the field anymore. Our policy is to do more transplants from living-related donors. We also want to increase the number of cadaveric organs we use. We are against commercialization. It is neither ethical nor humane.

Other physicians thought the root cause of the problem was the political tension between transplant centers, which prevented unified efforts throughout the country. The fragmentation caused by a lack of authority caused gaps that were filled by illicit deals between organ recipients, sellers, and the mafia. Yet all parties seemed to take organ trafficking for granted. It happened. While organ trade took root in the medical imaginary, the media was creating threatening images of predatory organ traders, "merchant" surgeons, the desperate poor, and the fortunate wealthy. Beyond the dark portrayal of transplantation by the media lay the striking dehumanization of patients and the decreasing value of living bodies. This kind of "positive eugenics" degraded whatever failed to fit in. Only the strongest would survive. The poor and destitute would have to live in an environment tainted by the naturalization of this worldview.

On the geographical plane, the areas of the country characterized by political instability and poverty became hot trading and smuggling spots for this practice: the southeastern region of the country, especially the border with Iraq, and also Istanbul itself, which was a bridge between Israel and Russia. As terrorists, freedom fighters, fundamentalists, prostitutes, pimps, engineers, soldiers, and merchants and dealers of all kinds moved across the region in response to capital, they merely added further layers to the violence of the underground trade in bodies. The new trade taking place in these zones was founded on the technology of unmaking and rebuilding the body. Its natural habitat was small private hospitals. At twenty years old, organ transplantation in Turkey had become a part of this landscape of bare and barren life;[74] it had become organ trafficking and the organ mafia. One of the transplant surgeons who described the large market of kidney and tissue trafficking from living donors believed that this was the part of the world where cultures and civilizations had risen, thrived, and faded away. Like some other physicians, he romanticized the ideas of civilization, progress, and the human while explaining people's relationship with science, technology, and progress in general. People who lived in this part of the world, now called the Middle East, were beyond civilization, he said; they had passed by this-worldly ambitions and gone back to a state distinctly different from what constitutes the modern and had done so by their own will, not by force. The Western neighbors and occupiers and the Western mentality had a hard time comprehending them: people who would not work for progress, maintain democratic regimes, or relate to life through modern means. (They did not want to control life; they were just in it. They could simply be with their *jann* and *nefes* [breath] and be complete as life took its course. This was a relationship with life.) People accepted, consumed, and appropriated anything they encountered, but all without planning, designing, or initiating. Despite their making use of ordered systems and mass production, they did not want to plan it. In a way they represented the point at which the West had failed to transform itself through techniques leading to neocolonialism, as the current war in the Middle East showed. Everything done in the name of progress and preserving life would fall apart because people had chosen to live apart from this-worldly concerns and closer to other worlds that resembled the imagined afterlife. In these places life hid behind barren mountains and in deserted villages, flowed through the wilderness of the Euphrates and Tigris rivers, and burned under the Mediterranean sun. It was full of invisible beings and forces—ghosts, jinn, terror, oppression, and many other *unknowns*—from within abandoned houses or beneath rocks and solitary trees.[75] Where systems of order failed, the boundaries between animal and human, terrorist and freedom fighter, death and *jann*, jinn and ghost, blurred.

There, the biopolis had acquired an invisible yet powerful aura through patients, physicians, and hospitals. Figures like the mafia, the gangster, the *eşkiya* (bandit), and the scandals of the organ mafia on private television channels, like heroic characters from folk tales made organ trafficking a major public issue in this aura. The resonance between images of the international mafia, conspiracy theories, and everyday violence enhanced the negative slant of these invented images. When a transplant patient in the mid-1990s traveled from Istanbul to Bombay, she was surprised to see so many patients from the eastern parts of the country on the same flight with her. Likewise, it had become common to have many transplant patients on board flights to Moscow.[76] One journalist could not forget his trip accompanying a transplant patient with IV tubes attached lying in the back of a shuttle bus all the way to Bağdat from Diyarbakır. Many similar surprises and life-transforming experiences awaited the transplant patients.

Despite its convenient congruence with this imaginary, organ trafficking was also a trade founded upon biomedical science. Its natural habitat was small private hospitals that more closely resembled mercantilist ventures than health-care providers like Aziz's metaphor of Moscow as an experiment. The rapid increase in the number of these boutique medical facilities in concert with that of private medical insurance companies and private laboratories was tainted by a background of rising unemployment and social inequality. In documentaries on scandals, TV cameras were zooming into the side streets of Istanbul to expose the malpractice and exploitation. Medicine was not recognizable in this form. It used to be that Turkish people traveled abroad to England, the United States, or Germany for superior health care. Scientific progress could not have changed so much as to make Turkey one of these temples of biomedical service. This could only be the "work of the mafia" as common sense ruled. This public assumption was enhanced by media broadcasts, everyday knowledge of how things worked in Turkey, and mistrust of local scientific research and medical progress.

THE BIOPOLIS'S VOCATIONS

Transplant patients went through stages of their treatment surrounded by physicians, nurses, and other health-care providers who at some point, in person or via hearsay, would become a part of their changing worlds. In this biopolis, technological objects were inventing vocations entangled not only in progressive high-tech medicine but also in mafia conspiracies or bone trade. These vocations were within the normalcy of social life, the ritual and the exchange; they were the "natural" actors of an economy of flesh and bones. Even though they operated between the legal and the illegal, the oppressor and the oppressed, the colonizer and the colonized, they were known as either criminals or businessmen: they remained within the normalcy of sociality. They lived upon segregation, poverty, or the vulnerability of the other. The deeply affectuous social transformations traceable in the life-less objects and in patients' psychotic experiences were the tools they depended upon. I encountered them almost on a daily basis, from little domestic corruption scandals in hospitals, which patients continuously complained about, to larger organizations that lived upon this changing neoliberal market and its easy unregulated ways. The organ mafia was one of its most popular symptoms.

The Organ Mafia

After the Berlin Wall came down in 1989 and the borders with formerly Communist neighbors opened, everyday life in Turkey took a different course. Many people in the region became mobile as trade routes opened. They traded diverse goods of various origins, shapes, and sizes in quasi-unregulated markets that emerged slowly. The organ trade became a hot subject for news reporters who wanted to expose the dark side of an emerging human trafficking of both labor and body parts. They began producing scandalous documentaries on organ trafficking in Istanbul and its links to Israel, Russia, India, and Iraq. The major producer of these images was an investigative program called *Arena*, which took on organ trafficking in a series of exposes.

> "Can I have a part of the money now?" asks the man. "I want to buy dresses for my two daughters before the holidays." The camera zooms in on the other man, Dr. S., a doctor in a green surgical gown.
>
> "Yes," says Dr. S. "I will give you $300 before the operation, and $3,000 after."
>
> "Will I recover quickly?" asks the man in a low tone.
>
> "Yes, in a few days you should be fine. And then you can spend some time with your family. Do not worry about your health my friend," Dr. S. replies reassuringly. "I am here, and I will take care of you. You just have to show up a day before the operation. Promise? Trust me. Look, everyone benefits from this: you can pay your debts and get your children back from your wife's parents, while saving the life of a poor Israeli who

has traveled all the way to Istanbul to find a kidney. She survives and you get your family back." *Cut.*

Three days later, late in the afternoon. Television journalist Uğur Dündar and a two-man camera crew walk through the front entrance of a private hospital in Istanbul. Dündar hurries down the white corridors. The camera follows him. *Cut.*

The camera zooms in on Dr. S., who has just come out of the hygiene room, his arms held upward to keep them sterile. In a slow-motion shot, he looks back and then turns around.

"Dr. S.!" Dündar yells. "Aren't you Dr. S.?" He continues, "Stop him! What are you getting prepared for? Who will you operate on? Hold him!" Dr. S. walks away and disappears in a crowd of nurses and hospital staff. The camera cannot catch him. *Cut.*

A shaky image back out in front of the hospital: Dr. S. is walking away from the building with another man—his lawyer. Dündar and the cameraman are running after him. "Admit it, Dr. S.!" shouts Dündar. "You were about to transplant a poor man's kidney into an Israeli patient. We talked to the patients. We set up a hidden camera a few days ago. We filmed the whole story. We got you, Dr. S. How much did you get this time? How much does the organ mafia charge for such operations?"

Dr. S. says nothing and walks away. *Cut.*

Back in the TV studio. "Aaaand . . ." begins the announcer, "Dündar has performed a public service yet again, and he caught the organ mafia as they were about to begin another illegal kidney transplantation. Dündar will always serve the welfare of the Turkish people and enlighten you. He will serve justice, no matter what!"[77]

In 1997 and 1999, *Arena* had broadcast two stories about Dr. S., the Turkish transplant surgeon who was conducting illegal kidney transplants between paid Turkish kidney donors and Israeli recipients. The segment described above had followed up on these cases.

The show had labeled Dr. S. the "organ mafia" and helped create the image of a Turkish underground medical community linked to international networks of crime. The episode's Faustian narrative framed characters from patients and doctors to dealers and donors as part of an evil engagement with the partly medical and partly commercial practice of organ trafficking. The characters were divided into clear categories of guilt and innocence.

The patients who went to mafia doctors seeking transplants were considered innocent because of their desire to survive. The donors who sold their organs were depicted as closer to evil because they compromised the integrity of their bodies. Dealers and the mafia physicians were depicted as the real criminals. The self-made Dr. S., with his close-cropped hair, diminutive figure, tanned skin, and frameless eyeglasses, looked more like a scientist character from an apocalyptic movie of the 1930s than a transplant surgeon. The scene of the crime and the criminals themselves were presented in this story as if they were marginal to the Turkish transplant community, as if illegal international kidney transplants were conducted by people who had no relationship to legitimate transplant practices in Turkey. But at the same time, the scandal was intensified because of catching an "organ mafia" "illegally" at work in a private hospital. This threatened the widespread public trust in good, "high-quality" and newly emerging private medicine. The figure of Dr. S. was at the center of the image of high-tech medicine in Turkey, where there had previously been little public awareness of scientific malpractice or experimentation on human subjects. Throughout the late 1990s, Channel D's *Arena* reporters continued their campaign to expose an organ mafia in Turkey and neighboring countries. One of the reasons they cornered Dr. S., they claimed, was to prevent the expansion of the illegal market in the country. But even catching him in the act was not sufficient evidence that he was committing a crime: his donors had signed consent forms, which proved voluntary action. What the journalistic sensationalism had achieved instead was to invent a distance between the "criminal/technological" and the "normal," between "transplants" and "medicine." This kind of renewed boundary between crime and ethics restored medical morality in a time of anomie and unemployment when Turkey was in deep financial crisis. "There is no such thing as the organ mafia in Turkey," said many physicians. There was not a single incidence of organ theft in the country, which would count as a "real" criminal act. They believed that transplanting organs with privately paid voluntary donors and recipients should not be seen as a crime but an ethical dilemma. To many Dr. S. was an unfortunate case of moral misconduct; he was simply unethical insofar as he was more or less open about the buying and selling of organs by those for whom he performed operations.

Over time, the broadcasted organ mafia scandals had given rise to the image of the immoral transplant physician, who was admired and surgically skilled. This had altered the image of transplants. Physicians were not as concerned about the quasi-illegal characteristic of the transplant pact between the bribed donor and the payee recipient as they were about the mafioso image transplants had acquired because of Dr. S.'s exposure. Nevertheless, with the same exposure they would discover the power of the media, and in time they would begin to use it for their own utilitarian and pragmatic ends. Transplants did become a "national thing" as this bond between the journalist and the transplant physician exalted to fix a broken self-image.

The organ trade in the Middle East seemed to follow paths similar to trade routes for opium, prostitution, and illegal migrant labor. Doctors like Dr. S. either engaged with dealers who would find potential donors themselves or with organ brokers, who mediated between physicians and donors. To the journalists who pursued Dr. S. it seemed more plausible that he had direct contact with the dealers who located potential organ sellers in the packed and smoky teahouses of Istanbul's slums. That is why they began their investigations there. In the Kasımpaşa district many unemployed people passed the time chatting about work, life, and politics or looking for work or for other ways of paying off their ever increasing debts. In such circumstances, selling a kidney was not out of the question; it was not *impossible*. The decision of the donor depended on the size and immediacy of his debts. It was the value of his body versus his family's destitution.[78] The journalists believed Dr. S. hired a few dealers—just like one would hire a cook, a driver, or a contractor—to approach these desperate men.

There were other donor groups besides the poor Turkish organ sellers. During her investigation of regional organ trafficking, the anthropologist Nancy Scheper-Hughes discovered immigrant workers from the same village from Moldova who had each sold one kidney to Dr. S. after arriving in Turkey for temporary construction jobs. Iraqi soldiers were believed to go to Adana, a place with a stable medical infrastructure in southeastern Turkey, to sell one of their kidneys. Turkish patients had been traveling to England, Russia, Iraq, and India since the mid-1990s for transplants. Israelis came to Istanbul to receive high-price transplants from Dr. S., and Dr. S. would fly to Ukraine, Italy, and Russia, where he would conduct multiple operations in a row at each location all with signed consent forms.

The chain that linked physicians and health-care providers to "dealers" and "bandits" was not arbitrary. Hospitals determined the flow of capital and the adaptation of legal language. In one hospital, dialysis patients were directed by their physicians to look into buying kidneys. At another hospital, maybe in another country, or another city, these same patients began second lives with purchased kidneys. Between many different hospitals lay continents, religions, health-care agents, drug companies, charter flights, travel agents, brokers, dealers, and objects of all kinds that hardly seemed to belong to medical practice in any traditional sense of the term. And in this unusual world, where *jann* was packed into single organs and transferred into other people's bodies, everyday relationships assumed a new form, and biomedicine was becoming just another ordinary business, with new values attached to its changing vocations.

The most famous face of this biopolis was Dr. S., who had begun his medical training at Istanbul University Medical School, where he pursued a career for a short while. He was then sent to Paul Brousse Hospital in Paris to learn transplant surgery. During his years in France, and then in Italy, he met many transplantation surgeons from all over Europe and the Middle East. Eurotransplant and the Middle Eastern Society for Organ Transplantation conferences served as platforms for networking, information exchange, and the forging of collegial friendships. One of the friends Dr. S. made this way was an Israeli physician who would come to send him many patients and also bring Dr. S. to Israel to operate. In the 1990s Dr. S. was transferred from Istanbul University Medical School to Haydarpaşa Numune Hospital and finally to Kartal SSK. He had conflicts with transplant surgeons and was caught doing illegal operations, which led to his being banned from public hospitals. He was no longer allowed to teach medicine, work in a public hospital, or pursue an academic career. But since the state could not actually rescind his medical degree, he could still continue his career as a transplant surgeon in private hospitals. From 1996 to 2000 he had operated on 360 patients, all with organs from donors who had given written voluntary consent. Only seven years later, one transplantation expert speculated, he must have operated on 2,000 people. This would constitute a quarter of all living related transplants in Turkey—the rough number of legal living related transplants in 2007 was approximately 6,000 people.

With his huge presence in the Turkish transplant community, Dr. S.'s name, face, and reputation became more than just the organ mafia, more than that of a simple criminal. Many Turkish physicians respected his surgical skills and the low mortality rate of his patients. Some patients called him "Robin Hood" because of his resistance to the elite Turkish medical establishment and his willingness to continue operating on patients despite his marginalization. Ironically, this Robin Hood was transplanting organs from the poor to the wealthy, a condition that had become "normal" within the naturalization of inequalities and the spirit of survival strategies.

Dr. S. was caught operating in different hospitals and released again. In 2002, he opened his own hospital. Over and over again he was caught conducting illegal operations on wealthy patients there. In May 2007, for example, Dr. S. was caught again after a gangster-like shoot-out in front of his hospital. A Turkish donor who had been promised U.S.$100,000 wanted more than the $2,000 advance he had been given before the operation. He came back to the hospital with a few friends, but since they were not allowed in a tense situation escalated, which turned into shooting in a short while. With the guns firing, the police arrived on the scene to find Dr. S. operating on two Israeli patients with Palestinian donors they had brought along. Both the recipients and the donors were being kept behind a locked door without doorknobs. When they were questioned by the police after being taken to a nearby hospital for care, both Palestinian donors insisted that their intentions were merely humanitarian. One praised the virtues of organ donation and said that as a Muslim he believed he would go to heaven if he saved a life. The other said he had sworn a vow after he was badly hurt in an accident that he would donate a kidney if he recovered. The Israeli and South African recipients likewise praised the voluntary consent of their donors. One was the former director of Israel's Organ Donation Foundation, the other a businessman. Dr. S.'s testimony was straightforward: he invoked the Hippocratic oath to "do no harm" and argued that these patients would have died had he not operated.[79]

The patients were sent to him by the same colleague in Israel with whom he had been collaborating for over a decade. The untrustworthy statements of all the parties involved in the story were as normal as Dr. S.'s reputation as Robin Hood. All of these contradicted people's lives and agency in the region and the world; they flew in the face of how those life stories were constructed and how heroes were made. Dr. S. was the central figure in this changing place of the body and its parts within a situation of inequality, social hierarchy, and authoritarian power. Rumor said he had surgery to change his own facial features so as to be unrecognized in public. And despite it all, he was still a member of the world transplant community, and there he was recognized as a skilled physician. And he continued working as a transplant surgeon as before: "I have worked in France, Italy, Germany, Ukraine, and Israel," he told me.

> Once, in Ukraine, I was invited to do a couple of transplants. I arrived there at night, and I went to the hospital to meet the doctors and nurses. . . . I had a great team working there for me. . . . Anyway, then I went to my hotel. In the morning I was driving to the hospital, I turned on the radio. Of course I did not understand the language; but I heard two words, "organ mafia," which were repeated over and over again. . . . At first I thought I was dreaming or mis-hearing. . . . But then they repeated it so many times; I thought there might be a trouble in the hospital. I called them on my cell phone. . . . They told me that the police had somehow been informed about the operations and they were looking for me everywhere. . . . I had to go directly to the airport and fly back home.

His voice grew louder as he described this adventure; but this would not stop him from doing transplants. He was merely working as a physician with donors who were donating voluntarily. As far as he was concerned he had become the scapegoat of the medical community, forced to confront the public each time journalists chased and caught him.

Dr. S. recalled accusations toward him when, in the midst of the earthquake emergency of 1999, the media began to alarm the public with headlines about the organ mafia. As the tension increased amid the destruction and the hundreds of aftershocks that followed the quake, these headlines caused more panic than the physical threats of natural disaster. While experts and politicians were trying to calm the public by denying the existence of an organ mafia, earthquake victims armed themselves against looters and organ thieves. This period of emergency saw the image of the organ mafia at its most potent and extreme. That fear of the organ mafia accompanied the fear of looting and violence at this time of national crisis was not surprising, however. Many unidentified bodies were taken to private hospitals, and with an official death toll of fourteen thousand people—much less than the number of people declared dead by Western NGOs—thousands of missing people could have been targets of the organ mafia.[80] That stressful time brought a new challenge to the label "organ mafia" for Dr. S.:

My thirteen-year-old daughter called me. She was on vacation with her mother in the south. She asked me if it was true that the organ mafia was kidnapping injured children for their organs. Can you imagine how I felt? My daughter was asking me if I was killing small children for their kidneys. But what else could she think? When they say "organ mafia" the first person who comes to mind is me. I told her that if I am the organ mafia—that is what people call me—if I am the organ mafia, then my child, I am telling you, I promise that no children and no human beings are being kidnapped or killed for a kidney.

Moreover, it is impossible to do any operations under such panic. Let us leave aside all the psychological pressure on the doctor; it is still impossible to do the tissue typing, to find the recipient, to find a crew, to find a place. Also, it is inhuman to think that a doctor is actually capable of pursuing such a difficult operation with the corpses of innocent people, just for money. I believe that the looters were mainly interested in kidnapping children. These looters are a big problem in Turkey, but the issue is always covered [by the media]. This time they put the blame on me.

Dr. Eldegez echoed Dr. S.'s assertion that the organ mafia could not be responsible for the large number of people whose families insisted they went missing after being rescued and sent to hospitals. Whatever the cause, literally hundreds of people lost their rescued family members and believed they disappeared in the hospitals. In the public imagination the peak of the tragedy was the fact that mass kidnapping and the exploitation of tragedy could be so coldly carried out by these underground body traders. The public was horrified by the "organ mafia" headlines, but at the same time somehow unsurprised. It was not inconceivable that those who had the power to organize underground crime would create an economy of bodies in times of political and social chaos and state emergency.

Yet, in general physicians shared Dr. S.'s views. There might have been a living-related organ sale in Turkey, but no surgeon who was skilled and educated enough to perform a transplant operation would be partner to murder for money. The living related kidney market was big and the number of donors was increasing day by day due to poverty; plenty of physicians were involved in it, but kidnapping and killing for organs required a totally different type of personality working with an immorality beyond comprehension.

The organ mafia became part of the formation of groups, religious and otherwise. Transplant surgeons recognized that there was a connection between European and Turkish organized crime, but Dr. S. was not involved with either of these groups. He was not engaged in criminal activity per se because he was not stealing organs; rather he was profiting indirectly from the sale of organs by being paid for performing operations for patients who would otherwise die. Thus he remained within the moral code of the Hippocratic oath. This kind of utilitarian liberalism flourished as markets opened to globalization and as vocations such as Dr. S.'s became potent and central forms of progress. This was an indication that violations of the human body, which, under fascism, would have seemed an extreme form of social Darwinism, were a natural fit with the ideals of development and progress of modern nations unable to maintain egalitarian social services. The mafia was a growing normalcy, a vocation in line with oaths and moralities, a defense against the bureaucracies imposed by the state and not a malignant abnormality. The nationalist politics that have been behind these structures became stronger and more legitimate with its growth. Patients were experiencing the "loss" amid these inequalities, as an underworld was becoming the legitimate ground upon which they or other patients began a new life.

The Bone Merchant

During the years in which the organ mafia became prominent in Istanbul, the novelist İhsan Oktay Anar published the novel *Puslu Kıtalar Atlası* (1995), which is set at a time when trade in human body parts was uncommon in the invisible shores of life in medieval Istanbul. Bünyamin, the main character, had become a dentist and a surgeon after studying the body parts he found dumped in the dark and wet streets of the ancient city; he was aided in his studies by books he got from traveling merchants and pirates. He was very careful that no one found out about the identity of the corpses he used for dissection: had the *kadı* (the judge) discovered he was using Muslim bodies as well as non-Muslim ones, he would have been in deep trouble.

Four hundred years later, Istanbul had changed a lot: human parts were now packed and labeled and sold as commercial products. Incarnations of Bünyamin were trading in the city openly. One such person was Ahmed, who traded in allografts—human bones used for orthopedic surgeries.

His company was on the main avenue of Beşiktaş, a business and trade district of the old Istanbul. The architecture of the neighborhood retained the dense aesthetic of a nineteenth-century Ottoman city—with narrow buildings that touched their neighbors on both sides like vertebrae in the spine and hung in a gentle curve over a hill to embrace the blue Bosporus. Ahmed loved the depth of his view toward the water. Situated so high up on this hill on the northern shores of the channel and the Marmara Sea, he felt as if he could see all the way to the Mediterranean. It drew him into thoughts of other lands, people, and cultures, and allowed a virtual journey into other lives. From this vantage, life seemed open and tolerant. Also for this reason, his location fit well into his business and his meetings with an American colleague who came to Istanbul for deliveries.

Ahmed had worked as a pharmacist in Ankara for many years before he began this new business in Istanbul. His company specialized in importing allografts, bone-grafting material, and was licensed to sell the products of a tissue bank based in the United States. Medical supply companies had been importing allografts since the 1990s. In the late 1990s and early 2000s, their profits grew greatly with the fourteenfold national increase in health-care expenditures. His business overlapped with the spirit that was dominant among generic drug producers back then, exemplified in the motto "*Hap yap, para kap*" (Make drugs, take [get] money). In all three import fields, generic drugs, allografts, and medical devices, many small- and medium-sized companies went into business. Bone grafts were in demand for operations to treat cancer, age-related conditions, and even traffic accidents. Physicians preferred allografts over metal implants because of the superior long-term results. Social security (both Emekli Sandığı and Sosyal Sigortalar Kurumu) covered the expenses of such operations. The demand was so high that Ahmed's company was planning on installing a second storage freezer at its office in Istanbul and importing even more bones from America.

While he believed that these products were of the best quality available on the market, Ahmed was also aware of the fact that competition was getting fierce. The allograft market had been expanding in recent years, and naturally Ahmed's company had competitors not just from the United States, but also Germany, France, and recently Belgium, as well as new bone traders from Bulgaria and Hungary. This new competition brought prices down. Ahmed was suspicious of the quality of the bones these companies used and the technology they had. These bones could carry viruses or other pathogens, or they could have been harvested without consent. It would not be hard to find human bones in the black markets of Eastern Europe, where almost everything had been traded since the fall of the Berlin Wall.

Nevertheless, to him it did not really matter where the bones originated as long as they were safe enough to be implanted. The American tissue bank Ahmed worked with was one of the leading tissue banks in the world; it produced freeze-dried bone grafts with sterilization steps that included 100 percent ethanol, gamma irradiation, and ethylene oxide treatments. Any virus would be erased by this screening. There were no proteins, "no life" left in them. They were lifeless, and no longer what they used to be, human.

As I sat with Ahmed in his office in Beşiktaş, it was raining outside, and an industrial fog settled in, obscuring the distant views. We could still see the luxurious Marriott Hotel across the street, hear the traffic, and smell the fog and exhaust through the windows. The heaviness of the city outside, as a background to our conversation, seemed to emphasize the tissue bank's status as a good Western friend, a well-armed chevalier coming to the rescue of Turkish patients. As we spoke, the American brokers and donors were closer to us than the Turkish people outside in the streets, who were running to seek shelter from the rain. It was one of those moments when the whole world shrank into the single word: globalization.

Globalization summed up the idea of business as if the global economy were an endless story. It also homogenized, universalized, reduced, and decontextualized economic processes. For example, Ahmed was uncertain about the origins of the bones with which he dealt. From what he heard, he believed they were harvested from African Americans and immigrant Mexicans in the United States. He and his colleagues even joked among themselves each time the American salesman came to Turkey with a load of bones for delivery. "How many Mexicans did you kill this time?" they would tease the salesman, and he would laugh with them.[81]

It was possible. Yet to a Turkish bone merchant, the imagined prior life of this economic practice was insignificant. It was only natural that Ahmed thought his bones came from illegal immigrants and the poor in the United States, from those who were powerless against the predations of global, high-tech biomedicine. The stereotyping was obvious but still striking. Ahmed also heard that bones were harvested from people in Nigeria. He qualified this information by describing it to me as hearsay. This story of the bones' origins, that there was something *behind* it, was not an urban legend to Ahmet; it was as real and as solid as the bones themselves. Whomever and wherever the bones came from, these people were long dead; the bones were screened, cleansed, and radiated. Along with the viruses in their blood, they had lost their human character, their identity; they had become "medical materials." There was nothing to be scared of about using them. Their origin, whether a poor Nigerian or a Mexican immigrant, was as absent as the syphilis, HIV, or Hepatitis B that might have infected them. Ahmed's main concern was about the reliability of the sources of bones others were importing.

The bone trade was only a thin slice of a global trade. Ahmed assumed Nigeria was a part of his business, but the occult dimension of that entanglement was not his concern. America, in Ahmed's imagination, was a supreme power that decontextualized bones, emptying them of humanity, transforming life into material by the use of reliable and safe high technology. It was Ahmed's trust in this safe American technology that kept the immorality inherent in acquiring and commodifying the bones separate from their legitimate and morally neutral economic value. Once the bones were in Turkey, it was as if they had lost all of their history and began a new life. They were categorized as "human-originating healing materials" (*insan menşekli iyileştirici malzeme*).

In the years to come, however, the Ministry would become aware of the abuse, corruption, and potential risks of the private bone trade and stop covering the expenses for allograft transplants. Many patients could not afford to pay for these expensive materials on their own, so physicians began using cheaper, artificial materials or autografts—the transplantation of the patient's own tissue—instead. Because of new regulatory controls, Ahmed had to close down his company: the demand for its products had radically decreased with the inflated prices. And so, during his few professional years in the biopolis, Ahmet was in the business of trading human bones. Then, he spent some time imagining the lives of those people whose bones were handed to him in the American salesman's bag, thanks to which he enjoyed an office with a view of the sea that gave him the feeling that he could see all the distant corners of the Mediterranean and from there to the world.

It was an open view.

TWICE INERT, LIFELESS AND LIFE-LESS

The self-imposed prohibition against harvesting bones in Turkey opened a door to the economy of bones for various tissue banks from all around the world. This quasi-human trade required new words and ideas to become a part of a natural practice. The universal term "graft" and the Turkish term "human-originating material" both were a part of this kind of a process of decontextualization. In orthopedic surgery bones were made into objects without biographies; their pasts were erased with radiation technology and screening; their identities were eroded. The substrate of the human person disappeared from them, diffused into a void so that they could become a mere structure, a lifeless object.

The treatment of the body as a thing that can be emptied out and re-filled via technology was analogous to discursive processes that disassociated the body from its kin to fill it with labor. Allografting technology was an example of this formation. In the eyes of the private medical supply firms, trading the body parts of others was merely a natural extension of market activity, one that was unconcerned with how these body parts were obtained. In the economy of grafts, the foreign bodies were radiated and cleansed of any pathogens, their bones becoming mere matrices for living patients all around the world, among them the people of Turkey. The imported grafts from foreign lands were in demand because of their *twice-inert* characteristic. In the patient's body and in the social body, they were *demineralized* objects with *assimilated* identities. They elided confrontation with the traditional flow of life.

Organ transplants were practiced in the same economy but with life-less objects: that is with objects that entailed familiarity and gave life—unlike the *lifeless* objects of the bone trade that entailed total alienation. In the invention and internalization of the life-less objects, the question of the *kadavra* prevailed. There were many naming efforts as there were with grafts: "brain death," "medical death condition," "last breath," all appeared as fleeting dark shadows that could only be seen in brief states of exception;[82] concepts which should fill the word representing the dead body as a life-sustaining entity. This kind of alienation of life from its former host for the social was hardly possible.

To understand this emerging universe of objects where *jann* was being fragmented and redefined to give a second life to transplant patients, I began tracing the word *kadavra* and its misgivings throughout the history of medicine in Turkey. In this history, I discovered a genealogy of life-less objects all stemming from efforts to utilize the human body for medical ends: the suicide, the insane, the cadaver, and the sacrifice. These were objects that were dead but somehow alive: in life, their personhood seemed to obscure the public, in death, they had acquired an exceptional status because of their obscured personhood in life. They were in part a challenge for medicine, including transplants, and in part for the collective life.

Like the *kadavra*, which had become transplant's foremost occupation throughout its thirty-year history in Turkey, these objects were used in rites of passage, in rituals, and in traditions to open and close relationships with life. In the historical genealogy of these *life-less* objects I found out about people marginalized, segregated, and discriminated against. Mainly their bodies could cease to be subjects to be transformed into technological objects, yet they were not entirely alienated. They had personhoods that could be restored anew so that they could become sociable objects utilized for medical ends in biomedical practices—and that with peace of mind.

As such, I saw a link between the *material invention* and the *local internalization* of such technological objects and patients' inner troubles, fears, and transferences during the transplant process. These objects were internalized and made local in the emerging universe where patients were being treated. Patients desired a continuity of life and a completeness of the body amid the uncertainties and alienation inherent in the histories of which they were involved.

This *affect* fragmented biopolitical agendas. It not only undid the political, economic, and legal categories with which I initially began my work on the commodification of the body, but it helped me look into other spheres of medicine and culture where I discovered the kin of these objects, which, traditionally, had invoked similar challenges for cultural life. These technological objects relied upon the same mechanisms of social life to become *twice inert* as other similar objects historically have. Through medical and social processes of elimination—through death and assimilation—human parts were made into bare objects with less life, so that they could be filled in with life through exchange. This way they could be internalized and made personal; this way they could be made one's own when taken in from the collective.

Patients' encapsulated experiences revealed this affect, this tension that was inherent in the making of objects from subjects, of things from people. It was an ontological process and an epistemological one. It was the dominant feeling in a hospital unit where transplant patients expected care and psychologically prepared themselves for a second life with a body part from another human being. And because it entailed such deep transferences, it was an explosion of meaning more than anything else. They felt they were facing something real about themselves as they related to *unknown* distant realities.

I continued my ethnography into spaces of death and histories of bare life to be able to interpret the undone meaning of life for these patients as they lived through high-tech or modern places. There, I not only found out about the *people*, but also about the initiating rites so that physicians and patients could make technology their own through basic economic processes. These rites and rituals were invented in spaces that were on the outskirts of social life. A dissection room was one of these settings, as were a mental hospital, an ICU, and a cemetery. In these spaces, people could live, die, or slide into another existence neither here nor there. I wanted to know the power of these spaces on transplant patients' lives for I could trace the affects of having a transplant operation to these settings through the way patients narrated their experiences via grammar, semantics, and rituals of their life histories. These discourses internalized the biopolis of Turkish medicine along with the reincorporation of the body, technologies, and social relations.

PART TWO

THE IMPOSSIBLE

SPACES OF DEATH

There is another city within Istanbul. Books call it
the "City of the Dead," a name hardly ever used locally in Istanbul. People know it as Eyüb Sultan, after
the *evliya* (saint) buried there.[1] It is the oldest Muslim cemetery in Istanbul. The tomb of Eyüb Sultan
is at the center of the cemetery, and it is surrounded
by mosques, tombs, and graves, which over the centuries have spread down the hill toward the shores of
the Golden Horn. It is as if they are almost piled atop
one another, half-standing and half-leaning, covered
with flowers and with grass growing equally wildly
all around. The scent of rose water poured on the
graves is said to invite angels as it mixes with the
sweet smell of pines in the breeze.

The legend of the City of the Dead is as unique
as the feelings it evokes. It dates back to the time of
the Ottoman conquest of Istanbul by the armies of
Fatih Sultan Mehmed. On June 1, 1453 CE, three days
after the conquest, Fatih Sultan Mehmed was having a conversation with Aksemşeddin, a feudal lord

who lived close to Istanbul whose troops had supported Fatih during the conquest. He told Fatih that he had seen a *nur* (a divine light) reaching into the night sky from the woods by the Golden Horn. Akşemşeddin believed that this *nur* belonged to Eyüb Sultan, the great warrior who fought in the army of Muhammad and then joined the armies of Muavviye to invade Constantinople, the capital of Byzantium. Eyüb was believed to have died in the war somewhere behind the city walls of Constantinople, and Akşemseddin thought he was providing a sign in the form of the *nur*, showing his tomb to the new Muslim rulers of Constantinople. Fatih decided to join Akşemseddin for a trip into the woods in order to see this sacred place, this place of *nur*. When they reached it, Akşemseddin picked two sticks from the ground and thrust them into the earth over where he believed the body of Eyüb Sultan lay, one over the head, the other over the feet, drawing a virtual line that symbolized the body. Fatih, however, was not truly convinced. After Akşemseddin left, Fatih gave his royal ring to his guard and told him to bury the ring between the sticks and then to place the sticks somewhere far away. The next day Fatih asked Akşemseddin to join him in another visit to Eyüb Sultan's place of death. When they arrived, even though the sticks had been removed, Akşemseddin pointed to a spot on the ground over Eyüb's dead body and told Fatih that his ring was buried there. Fatih came to believe that this was indeed the sacred place where Eyüb Sultan had been killed. Akşemseddin had proved his wisdom and intuition by discerning the trick Fatih had attempted to play on him, and so Fatih ordered the construction of a *türbe* (a saintly tomb) on the site.

As centuries passed, *türbe*s for many more important figures—such as Sokollu Mehmet Pasha, the prime minister to Süleyman the Magnificent, and Ali Kuşcu, the famous mathematician—were built around Eyüb's tomb, and so the cemetery became known as the City of the Dead. Sultans' wives and children were also buried there in separate *türbe*s among pasha families, doctors, and locals from the neighborhoods surrounding the Golden Horn. The name City of the Dead reflected the liveliness of death: it was a city where life continued invisible to the eye of the worldly people but parallel to it and *known* by the heart. It was a city that opened a connection with the world after this, and thus all important Muslim rituals were institutionalized there. One could say prayers and sacrifice animals; one could shop for holy books at the entrance, have a cup of tea on the hills above, and walk the pleasant trails amid the woods and tombs; one could think about life and the meaning of salvation. Many ill people visit the City of the Dead, believing that their petitions will be received sooner if they pray *El-Fatiha* for the salvation of Eyüb's soul.[2]

This cemetery became *known* as the place where the healing power of Eyüb's *nur* could be felt. The light that shone through the green glass decorating Eyüb's tomb and reflected off the surfaces of the ancient blue tile mosaics—unique pieces of art that cover the walls of the tomb and the mosque—is said to be Eyüb's *nur* sheltered by the two sticks that now have grown into enormous trees shading the courtyard during hot summer days. The *nur* of Eyüb Sultan is at work everywhere: in the tomb and the mosque, in the trees and in the water. Visitors line up to say *El-Fatiha* for Eyüb Sultan and whisper their vows to him. When they come out of his tomb and into the courtyard, they drink the sacred water that springs from under the two trees in the hope of benefiting from its healing powers.[3] The Diyanet has put up official signs just above the fountains: "This water does not heal," "Expecting healing from water is superstitious and is against Islam," and other such warnings—as a call for reason. Despite these signs, children, women, men, the ill and the healthy continue to fill their bottles with the sacred water to make this divine light ignite their own vitality with each sip.

The gravesite was considered sacred long before Eyüb by the local orthodox Christians in the Byzantine period that preceded Fatih's conquest. They would come to these woods to pray and to drink from the springs, which they too believed had sacred healing powers.[4]

Walking to Eyüb Sultan down Pierre Loti Hill—named after the French writer and traveler who lived and worked there in the late nineteenth century—and looking past the half-standing, half-leaning gravestones to the blue waters of the Golden Horn and the ships from all around the Mediterranean sailing to the Black Sea beyond, one can easily lose track of time. The walk evokes serenity, a move through endless time and imagined spaces. Likewise, the City of the Dead is actually a metaphor to remind people of the eternal dimensions of human life. In Eyüb Sultan, the dead speak to the living from the gravestones, connecting them with the invisible realms of infinity. One of the *hodja*s in Eyüb Sultan says that one must heal human beings spiritually as well as medically.[5] He says human beings can only find salvation in the *idealistic lives* of those who have become models for salvation and healing. It is hard to find such souls, though they inhabit Eyüb Sultan and similar tombs in Anatolia. Saints in particular, with

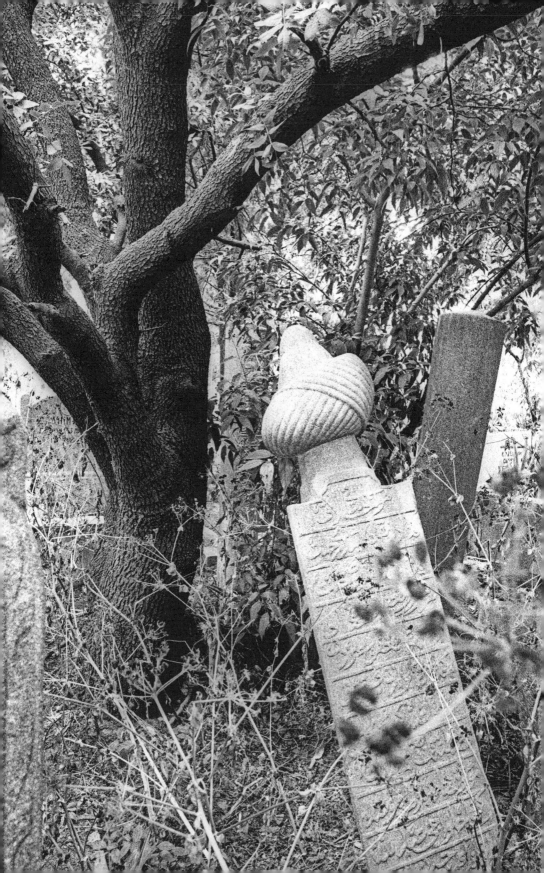

their pure and sacred presence, he says, connect the living with life in the hereafter.

The City of the Dead speaks for itself. It represents the life of the dead and the unboundedness of the human spirit in space and time. Illness and healing are central to this space. They hasten or slow the passage of the living across the boundary between the world and the afterlife, giving rise to a heightened consciousness of one's being. For many it is a space where self-understanding can take shape.

Life in the cemeteries—the blossoming flowers, stray cats, trees leaning over graves, and people visiting the deceased every day with joy and care, as if visiting a museum filled with their own belongings—all these evoke an existence from one form to another, the transformation of active living to resting in the cemetery. The cemetery phase of human life is said to end only with resurrection on Kıyamet, the Day of Judgment. Oral tradition and Qur'anic verses suggest that on that day Dabbet-ül Arz, a winged creature with the face of either a human or a cow, pig's eyes, elephant ears, a horse-like body, and human hands, will come out of the earth and rank all humans.[6] As in Christianity, life in this world is seen as a preparation for eternal afterlife. Resurrection, an indispensable aspect of Islamic cosmology, is the final birth into an eternal life to be spent either in heaven or in hell.

In the Qur'an,[7] the events of human history, both individual and collective, are in the hands of a just and merciful God, and death is not the end but the passage into a new and eternal existence.[8] Verses about the day of resurrection symbolize the irrelevance of human life on Earth, stressing its shortness in comparison to eternity: "'How many years did you stay on the earth?' They say: 'We stayed one day or a part of it. Ask the accountants,'" says the scripture (Qur'an 23:112–13). Cosmological space, not astronomic time, is thus the more significant measure of human life. All of human history moves from the creation to the eschaton. Signs such as the Dabbet-ül Arz precede the Final Judgment, signaling the arrival of the final hour.[9] The individual life cycle plays out within this overall structure of creation: birth, death, and resurrection. In Qur'anic narratives, birth, death, and resurrection structure life in Muslim cosmological space.[10]

---

1. "Eyüp 2" by Laleper Aytek. Courtesy of the artist.

In this cosmology, the dead body begins a new life in the cemetery as it decays in the earth. The decomposition of the dead body does not mean that the corpse loses its human shape, the mirror image by which, according to the Qur'an, the self knows its own constant self-similarity: "Did they not see that God Who created the skies and the earth is powerful to create the same of them, and make them a time? No doubt about it!" (Qur'an 17:99). God, having created each human once, is able to re-create the same being. This identical mirror image rises from the earth in its completeness despite having decayed in the grave for centuries. This is the main underlying idea behind resurrection: the *resurrection of the self*. The body in its worldly appearance represented this transcendent and enduring self-image. Conversely, this imagined self-image is the only way to know oneself.[11]

The Qur'an contains vivid verses concerning the body, its image, its creation, and its resurrection:

O People! If you are in doubt about the resurrection, surely We created you from a soil[,] then from a drop, then from a clot, then from a formed and unformed live flesh in order We to explain to you [*sic*]. We settle in the wombs whom We wish up to a fixed time. Then We extract you as a baby. Then you reach your age of full strength. Some of you are caused to die, and some of you are returned to the feeblest old age, so that they know nothing after they knew. You see the earth barren and lifeless. But when we send down on it the water, it stirs and swells and puts forth every kind of beautiful herbage. [Qur'an 22:5]

Then we transformed the clot into the lump, and transformed it into the bones. We dressed the bones with a meat-flesh. Then we generated it into another creation. So glorification be for God Who is the best Creator! [Qur'an 23:14]

Does the human being think that We shall not gather his bones?
Yes! We are able to make him complete[,] even his very fingertips.
[Qur'an 75:3–4]

Qur'anic resurrection narratives are understood by many believers to tell the history of the body, the remaking of rotten bones and the growth of flesh over these bones like water bringing life back to the lifeless earth. The resurrection of the self with the self-identical body also reconstitutes the memory of the past life. The dead body will rise from its grave a complete being, put back together by God, all of its parts intact and perfect.

This idea of resurrection shaped burial practices: the dead were not buried in coffins because their bodies should be able to rise up from the ground without having to break out of a box. Traditionally the body was washed in the mosque by the deceased's relatives immediately after death and placed in a coffin, which bearers carried to the cemetery on their shoulders. Final prayers were said around the grave, and the body, wrapped in a long white shroud, was removed from the coffin and placed in the grave to the accompaniment of further prayers around the grave, which might include a headstone. While the body decayed in the shroud, the *shape of the shroud* traced the lines of the *body's original image*. At the resurrection this form would be filled with flesh again.

Life in the cemetery is a life of anticipation of the Hour, organized around a unique relationship between imagination and reality and a specific cultural attitude toward death. The imagined spaces of the cemetery and the afterlife are as real as this world. Because space predominated over time as a defining factor of this cosmology, when dead bodies were moved from this positively valued space to some other place, a whole worldview was put into question. The biopolis embodied an experience in the shift of the notion of space in this sense.

In the high-tech age, as new concepts of death and dying emerged in hospital settings, the culture of death only became troubling for a proper medical practice, as in the attempts to gain acceptance for the category of a brain-dead donor with a beating heart, commonly referred to as a *kadavra*. Historically, however, the first such interruption to life cycles in spaces of death was with regard to anatomy, wherein the word *kadavra* was introduced as a Turkish adaptation of the English *cadaver*. With transplantation technology, transplant surgeons began using the same word for the brain-dead donor.

Given the continuing metaphysical, ritual, and meditative life in cemeteries, both transplantation and anatomy dissections made the hospital and the laboratory cemetery-like spaces for donated dead bodies. Anatomists retained bodies for a long period of time, postponing the burial for one to two years. When these bodies were returned from these spaces for burial, they either lacked organs or had been sliced to pieces. Dead bodies in such conditions were unacceptable and a challenge to the self-image and ideals of Turkish doctors themselves, who had to transform death and dying in the midst of their efforts to maintain Western-style high-tech medicine and medical education.

THE POOL OF THE DEAD

> And then there is the pool of the dead. It is a place only a few know of. And only with strict permission, one is allowed to see it. They dump the dead bodies of the mentally ill there to use them for dissection.
>
> —DR. OSMAN, *a brain surgeon at Bakırköy Mental Hospital*[12]

As was also the case in Europe in the nineteenth century and the early twentieth, it was difficult to obtain cadavers for medical training and research during Turkey's early modernization in both the Ottoman and Turkish republic periods. At the old Ottoman buildings of Haydarpaşa Medical School, I was told that it was so hard to find corpses to use for anatomical research in the Ottoman era that students were rumored to have dug a tunnel from the school to a nearby graveyard in order to secretly gather them. I was shown a virtual path that was supposed to follow their underground passage to the graveyard of *Ga'yrimüslim* (non-Muslims).[13] Anatomical dissection was legalized in 1841 by Sultan Mahmud at the urging of a Viennese physician, Dr. Charles A. Bernard, who initiated research and instruction in pathology at the Mekteb-i Tıbbıye Şahane, the first modern medical school in the empire. It is said that the sultan agreed to pass the Dissection Act on the condition that only the bodies of non-Muslims be dissected and Muslim bodies not be violated. While religious identity was at the center of this discourse of *difference*, unlike the Body Act of 1832 in England,[14] bodies of the poor and the homeless were not allowed to be used for dissection in the Ottoman Empire.[15]

With the rise of the Turkish republic in 1923 and the continuing modernization of medical education in the 1930s and 1940s, physicians had to find supplies of cadavers for the increasing number of medical students. Medical instructors could not force people to donate their relatives' dead bodies; donations should be made naturally out of a sense of social solidarity and service to the public good of medical advancement. In the early days of the republic, faith in the natural flow of modern life and urban organic solidarity was the dominant mode of thinking. Social reformers and followers of

Atatürk believed that the modern division of labor would give rise to a new form of organic social solidarity. They embraced the view of Durkheimian thinkers such as Ziya Gökalp (1876–1924), who argued that modernity would unfold naturally out of more traditional mechanical solidarity systematically driven by individual will and action.[16] However, the modernizing reforms were still young. The medical education system's need for research materials could not await the natural "flow" into organic modern unity. Physicians required real corpses for their anatomical research. In their search for a practical solution to this problem, they turned to another sphere of medical care, the mental hospital, as was common practice in England at the time.[17]

In a move that tells us a great deal about the value of "normal" dead bodies, the medical community decided to use unclaimed bodies of the mentally ill from the state hospitals for dissection. The law had granted doctors the right to appropriate dead bodies of the homeless for dissection. But it was hard to find homeless people in sufficient numbers anywhere other than in mental hospitals. In villages, families took care of each other. In cities like Istanbul, urban immigrants built homes in little *gecekondu* (slums) in the suburbs of the city. As a result, there were not many homeless people. Even though the police were required by law to inform anatomists when a homeless person was found dead on the street, they would typically inform the person's extended family and ask them to pick up the body instead. Only on the rare occasion when a homeless person died in the emergency room of a university hospital would the anatomy lab would be informed.

Instead of trying to get the police to change their practices, doctors turned to mental hospitals. The institution at Bakırköy was a potential cadaver source because of the increasing numbers of patients abandoned there. From the 1930s onward, many families from remote parts of Anatolia brought mentally ill relatives to this hospital in Istanbul. In most cases, patients were left at the hospital and their families never returned for them. By the early 1950s the hospital was overflowing with these abandoned people. The years after the Second World War were difficult times. Despite Turkey's noninvolvement in the war, this economically and politically unstable period was marked by poverty and increased migration from villages to big cities. Villages had emptied out as rural people were drawn to the promise of wealth in Istanbul. But labor migration came with a price. Families could no longer afford to take care of their mentally ill relatives, and more and

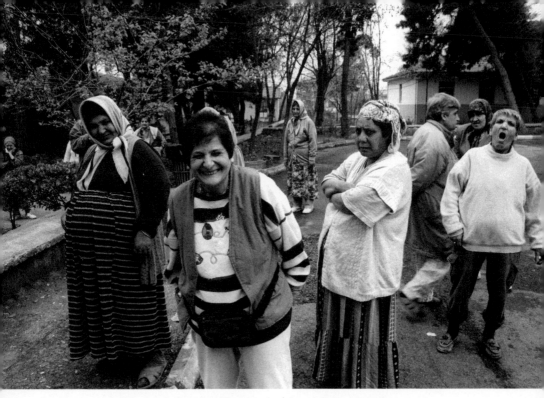

2. Patients at the Bakırköy Mental Hospital. "Bakırköy 1" by Laleper Aytek. Courtesy of the artist.

more of them were delivered to Bakırköy Mental Hospital. Mercy had vanished from the life of the small industrializing family.

Though this practice was common knowledge among medical students, it was not publicly known. It was not something physicians were proud of or a topic that they liked to discuss. It was typically spoken of as a tragic consequence of miserable conditions in the health-care system in general, a sign of the poverty of hospitals and a misgiving of Turkish medical education. When an orthopedist described to me how he learned dissection at Istanbul University's medical school in the early 1980s, I had already heard similar stories on the subject related in a similarly melancholic tone. "I think it was because it was right after the military putsch on September 12, 1980," he told me. "I was a student at the medical school; it was a time of tension and political upheaval. Life was restricted, and for that reason, we had to learn dissection on the corpses of the schizophrenics and the abandoned that were delivered to us from Bakırköy Mental Hospital."

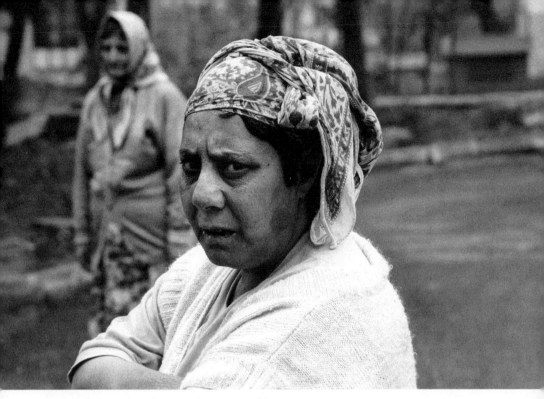

3. "Bakırköy 2" by Laleper Aytek. Courtesy of the artist.

The corpses did come from the mental hospital, but the military putsch was not the reason why medical students had to learn dissection on the bodies of the mentally ill. The difficulty of finding cadavers for research, the cultural privileging of the deceased's repose in the cemetery, and the mass abandonment of the mentally ill all combined to encourage the use of these latter bodies in anatomy. The anatomists had made an arrangement with Bakırköy Mental Hospital to have the bodies of the abandoned delivered for preservation in the *ölü havuzu*, the pool of the dead, an old swimming pool filled with a solution of formaldehyde in the basement anatomy lab at Cerrahpaşa Medical School. If within six months family members came to retrieve the body, it would be returned to them. Otherwise it would be used for dissection.

In Turkey, mentally ill people were denied full legal personhood because of their dependence and mental health. They had no rights over their own bodies. If their dead bodies were not claimed from the anatomy lab then they were also regarded as homeless. Because of the miserable conditions

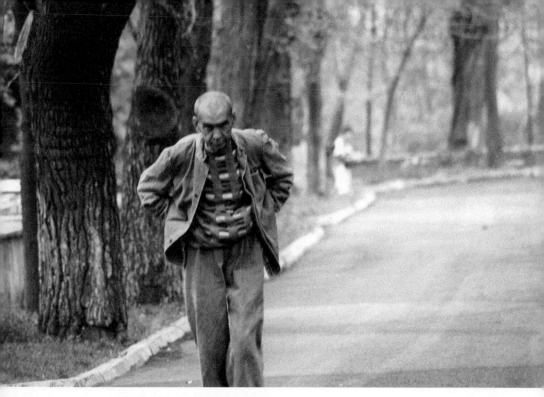

4. "Bakırköy 5" by Laleper Aytek. Courtesy of the artist.

of life in the mental hospital throughout the early years of the republic, many of these patients died of epidemics or malnutrition. They provided the medical school with sufficient cadavers for dissection until the 1980s— after the most recent coup—when the number of medical students increased dramatically. Even after the significant improvements made by Minister Yıldırım Aktuna's reforms back in the mid-1980s, conditions in the mental hospitals were very poor. Many patients shared very small rooms and slept in beds that almost touched one another (a condition that still persisted in the early 2000s), they received food once a day, and they did not have proper clothes. Under these conditions, many died. After death, their bodies became available for medical purposes—"serving society," as one anatomist told me.

MEHMED

Mehmed lay on the operating table. His skin now as brown as the earth itself, he had been delivered to the anatomy lab almost a year ago. A young assis-

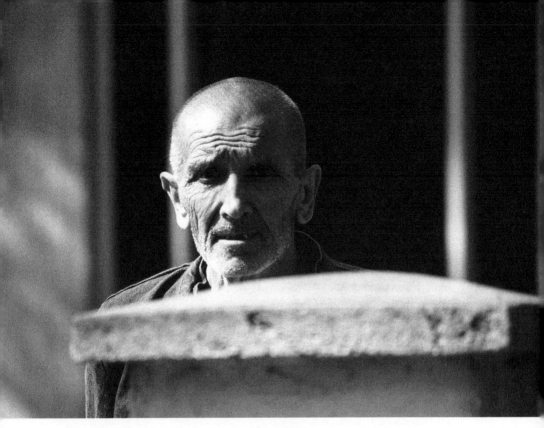

5. "Bakırköy 6" by Laleper Aytek. Courtesy of the artist.

tant anatomist showed me how his body had been dissected. The doctors referred him to as "Number 85," replacing his real name during what they called his new "transitional phase" in the lab. He had another number at the mental hospital, where doctors referred to him as 564/2956. Still, the dead body had a name: Mehmed.

Mehmed was born in the year 1337 of the Islamic calendar—1921 according to the Medeni Takvim, the Roman calendar, which was implemented in Turkey not long after his birth.[18] Mehmed lived with his family in the village of Kayalar, near Edirne, a city that was the capital of the Ottoman Empire until the conquest of Istanbul. He had worked as a *rençber* (laborer) in Kayalar, weeding farmers' crops and chopping wood. Mehmed's father died when he was young. His mother remarried in order to be able to take care of him and his sister, who was mute. It was before this marriage, however, in 1946, that Mehmed was first sent to the mental hospital in Istanbul, for reasons that are not clear—no record was kept on his first visit. It could have been distress related to the tragedy of his father's death, or to the new family and his mother marrying another man. He remained at the hospital for a few years, until his new stepfather came to Istanbul to bring him back. Mehmed came back to Kayalar and helped his stepfather farm the land he owned. His mother had become pregnant shortly after the second marriage, and their family was growing.

Mehmed lived with his family for seven more years, until one day his stepfather brought him to the police department with a request to deliver him back to the mental hospital. "He is showing violent tendencies," his stepfather claimed. "He is aggressive, he attempted to kill his niece, he does not talk to anyone, he does not understand what is said to him." Two days later, Mehmed was delivered to the Bakırköy Mental Hospital in Istanbul. It was November 14, 1953. Thirty-two-year-old Mehmed was examined for a mental illness that might have caused his aggression.

In his first meeting with his doctor, Mehmed did not utter a word. When the doctor asked if he had a mother, Mehmed nodded his head slightly in response. To the question of whether he had a father, he shook his head no. He began receiving electroshock therapy: 300 watts for one-and-a-half minutes at a time.

In a second meeting a few days later, the doctor asked Mehmed if he knew where he was. He made an anxious face and would not answer. When the doctor asked him if he was ill, he did not utter a word, but he shook his head no. The doctor asked Mehmed why his family had brought him to the hospital. Mehmed began to shiver but could not answer. "Are you feeling discomfort?" the doctor asked him. Mehmed shook his head. "Do you hear voices out of nowhere?" He shook his head. "Do you have *hayal* [visions]?" He shook his head. The doctor asked if Mehmed thought he had enemies, and again he shook his head. What else could the doctor ask him before he could make a sound diagnosis? The objective questions. He asked him what year it was. Mehmed looked at him, puzzled. What month was it? He did not respond. The doctor noted that he had been admitted to the mental hospital because he reportedly behaved violently toward his mother and stepfather, that he had been diagnosed with a mental illness characterized with abnormal social behavior. The doctor reported in his notes, "He does not speak to anyone, does not show any reaction to his environment, eats little, does not sleep much, and he does not rape."

A year later, the diagnosis schizophrenia appeared in Mehmed's file. He still did not speak to anyone, but he continued to receive electroshock therapy in accordance with the hospital's routine treatment for acute aggressive cases—therapy every day for the first two weeks of residence at the hospital. When patients felt better, the dosage was reduced.

Four more years passed. Life in the hospital was miserable, but the patients, due to heavy medication, might not have realized the misery of their abandonment. Like Mehmed, most of the patients were brought there by their families from faraway villages in Anatolia. Istanbul was the big city, and its streets were believed to be paved with gold. The mental hospital was the uncanny place that provided a solution to migrant families whose relatives were troubled, behaving strangely, and not speaking to them. This was how Mehmed and many like him were abandoned at the hospital over decades. Time stopped for them the moment they passed through the high walls of the gardens that surrounded it.

Mehmed started talking to himself at last, the doctor reported. And once he might even have spoken to or communicated in a rather clear way with the doctor, as there is a report in Mehmed's file that the doctor was concerned that he may have been raped by a male nurse.

Eight years after Mehmed's arrival in the hospital, without a single visit from his parents, his stepfather went to court to withdraw Mehmed's right of citizenship, thereby denying him freedom of movement. In June 1961, the court ruled that due to his unstable schizophrenia, Mehmed's citizenship was to be withdrawn and guardianship given to his stepfather. Mehmed was then forty years old. He lived in a place with people like himself; he ate well, slept well, did not talk to anyone, walked up and down the garden all day long, did not care about his environment or his personal hygiene, and did not rape. This was his medical record for the forty years of his life. The hospital gardens, built over an ancient Byzantine necropolis, and the other chronic patients there were all the world and society he would know for the rest of his life.

The mental hospital was one of the poorest hospitals in the country, not least because of the lifelong bed service it offered to abandoned patients. If families did not leave the right phone number or address and did not come to see their relatives, the hospital would send the police to find them and force them to visit. Thirty years after his arrival at Bakırköy, when Mehmed was sixty-two years old, the hospital administration sent a request to the police in Kayalar to find his parents and send them to come see their son. They received no answer. Almost ten years later, the hospital tried again.

In October 1994, administrators finally received a police report that both of his parents and his siblings had died. Only one of his cousins, who lived in Istanbul, was alive. In 1998, as Mehmed suffered from a long-standing lung problem, the doctors decided to contact his cousin. The cousin refused to visit, saying simply that all of Mehmed's family had already passed away.

On January 19, 2000, a woman from Mehmed's unit died; like Mehmed's sister, she was mute and she had been at Bakırköy since 1957, shortly after his own arrival there. At the end of that same year, on December 13, Mehmed collapsed just as he was standing up from the lunch table after finishing his meal. A nurse who was present, who had known him a long time, could not tell what was wrong with him. Worried about a heart attack, she sent an anxious note to the emergency room to have him examined. The next morning at 6:45 AM, suffering from a heart attack, Mehmed closed his eyes and died in the mental hospital where he had spent fifty years of his life. He had no one.

Four days passed. The hospital's administrators requested that the anatomy lab preserve the body of this homeless person who had died in the hospital, and two days later they delivered him to the anatomists. It was then that his brief new life "in the service of humanity" began. For a second time Mehmed was assigned a number, and then he was placed in a pool of preservative chemicals that would tint his flesh an earthen color.

Six months later, when the official waiting period after informing his family of his death had elapsed, Mehmed was laid on a surgery table in the anatomy lab dissection room. His eyes were open. His head hung and fell back. I looked at him. I had not yet read his file—I did not know who he was. There was another body lying next to his—one the anatomist described as "too fat" to properly dissect. It was the body of a mute patient, a woman who was delivered to Bakırköy shortly after Mehmed, and had died one year before him. She lay next to him in silence like a sister in confinement and in death.[19]

I gazed at them still, standing between the two beds.

INSANITY

In Turkey, the cultural understanding of mental health is rather complex. In the Sunni Muslim tradition, insanity is not narrated as something evil

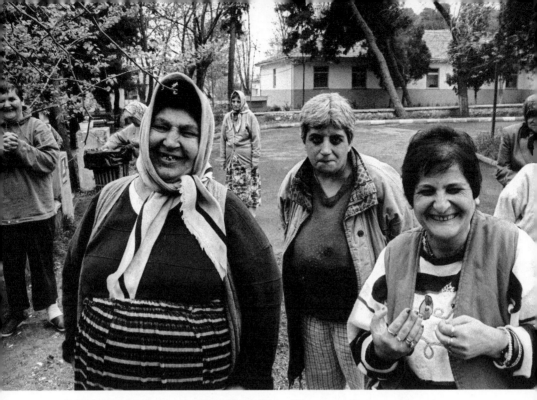

6. "Bakırköy 3" by Laleper Aytek. Courtesy of the artist.

or monstrous, nor do people view the mad as a threat.[20] Insanity is more like a categorical mark of difference in human beings' creation by God. The category of mental normalcy is articulated through and against the category of insanity.

During the Ottoman era, prior to the establishment of modern mental hospitals in Istanbul, the mentally ill were treated in a *bimarhane*, a place of healing, which later became known as *tımarhane*, a place of discipline.[21] But as they were established, these *tımarhanes* were not as ambiguous as the mental hospital would be as an iconic space of exclusion in Istanbul's modern life. Popular plays depicted *tımarhanes* within the communal life back in the nineteenth century. Likewise the Turkish Karagöz shadow play *Tımarhane*, one of numerous traditional plays featuring the recurring characters Karagöz and Hacivat, depicted madness as a part of daily life: as something that can happen to anyone, as an inherent feature of being human, and as a product of social life embodied in the *repetition of words*.[22]

In the first act of the play *Tımarhane*, Karagöz is walking in his own neighborhood in Istanbul when he meets a man who speaks to him in

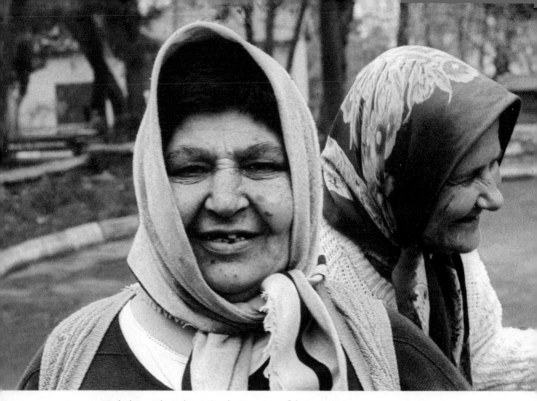

7. "Bakırköy 4" by Laleper Aytek. Courtesy of the artist.

nonsense. Karagöz ignores him, but a few minutes later, he meets another man speaking in a similar fashion, and soon after, a third one. Just as Karagöz begins to get angry at these men because he cannot understand them, he meets Hacivat, the wise character who appears in many plays and uses his wits to rescue Karagöz from trouble. Hacivat suggests they ask the people of the neighborhood if they think these mad people should be sent to the *tımarhane*, and the locals all agree that they should.

In the second act, Karagöz meets one of the insane men on the street again and gets very angry. In his anger, however, he begins to talk like them.[23] Seeing that Karagöz has become insane like the others, Hacivat decides to take him to the *tımarhane* along with the three others, where they are all put into chains. Eventually, the three insane men escape their chains and flee the *tımarhane*, but poor Karagöz is left there alone and in chains. Hacivat pities Karagöz, who is unable to get out of the situation on his own, so he calls for the European doctor to examine him. The doctor starts asking Karagöz questions. Even though Karagöz answers the doctor incorrectly at first, he soon manages to give the right answers and is liberated from his chains.

This play is almost a microcosm of the historical and cultural development of the early understanding of the mental hospital in Turkey where insanity was viewed as an infectious condition in which abnormal speech caused its like—if one lived with the insane one would become like them. The popular idiom "*Körle yatan şaşı kalkar*" (One sleeping next to the blind wakes up cross-eyed) reflected a parallel idea; likewise, Oğuz's depiction of his sessions with a therapist and the other patients he saw there was rooted in this idiom's affect. Thus in the nineteenth century, the insane were imprisoned in *tımarhane*s in part to discipline their speech. Controlling their words meant controlling norms and consequently controlling the body.

While today people do not ridicule or harm the mentally ill in their neighborhoods, the mental hospital is regarded as an isolated island within Istanbul. As in Karagöz's *Tımarhane*, it is not insanity itself but the *space of the insane* that is viewed as foreign and dangerous to the normalcy of everyday life and brought to an extreme by the exclusion of the mental hospital from city life through the use of high walls. It is characterized by repressed social issues, political violence, and failed humanity. It represents all those that were and had been kept from public sight. This space, like few others, had become an asylum for the poor and the excluded,[24] where people like Mehmed lived in a state of abandonment as modernity institutionalized the uncanny by keeping them apart, by segregation.

As a part of the history of the mental hospital, Dr. Osman, a brain surgeon in Bakırköy, told me the story of a few patients' attempts to escape in the 1930s. In response, Bakırköy's physicians posted news of the escape in the local newspapers to warn the public. (Mehmed's file indicates his own attempt to escape in the late 1960s.) Such warnings, Dr. Osman thought, portrayed mental patients like criminals who had just escaped from prison. A public anxiety about Bakırköy started developing with this "escape" discourse in the 1930s. In the novel *Saatleri Ayarlama Enstitüsü* (1962), by Ahmet Hamdi Tanpınar (1901–62), the modern mental hospital is a central space where Western science would be made local through psychoanalytic and other processes and its image is that of a modern place one had to escape to remain human. To speak of the way Turkish people feel torn between East and West, Tanpınar introduces the physician as the central element that transformed the space from *tımarhane* to a prison-like asylum.

He writes of the therapies of a Freudian psychologist who took charge of a patient and began one of the first psychoanalytic treatments in the country with him. The patient gets very disturbed by the sessions, and the physician gets upset by the fact that the patient cannot even dream properly so as to be able to make psychoanalysis possible. During a visit at the hospital the patient's wife asks him to begin dreaming according to the symbols the Vienna-trained physician understood, so that the physician could interpret the patient's dreams and in time release the patient from his imprisonment there.

In the era after the Second World War, the mental hospital had already transformed the semiotic place of insanity beyond the illness of individuals and beyond God's sign of difference. The dark space of the hospital, in which insanity exceeded a traditional understanding of abnormality, was taking on a meaning in itself as a space alien to society at large. The insane were no longer tangible examples that proved the value of sanity. The modern space overdetermined the life of the people who began inhabiting it.

When physicians from the mental hospital told me about how life outside was much more dangerous than theirs inside the hospital, they were speaking of this kind of alienation created by the space. Physicians told me how free they felt among the insane. In contrast to its stigmatized image, for physicians Bakırköy was the place where they practiced their vocation. It was the place with which they identified despite its cultural stigma. "People believe that we are all mad here," one said as we were having tea in the hospital's courtyard. Twice, men had approached and asked for cigarettes, and they were invited to join us. "They [society] try to make us invisible," continued the psychiatrist. "Nobody wants to deal with these poor people. They are okay. We share the same coffee shop, drink our tea together, smoke together. They have no one, they are abandoned. We are like a big family here. Anyway, they would not do any harm to anyone. People out there," he pointed out to a place through the gardens and beyond the high walls, "they are the real danger, they are unpredictable."

KADAVRA

Cerrahpaşa Medical School, home of the anatomy lab where Mehmed was delivered upon his death, is located in Beyazıt, an old district on the European side of Istanbul. Built on the shores of the Bosporus, Cerrahpaşa had been a part of Istanbul University Hospital until its establishment as an independent entity in 1969. In its Ottoman buildings next to the medical school's new architecture and surrounded the ruins of Byzantine city walls, nineteenth-century surgeries were performed.

Patients line up in front of different medical units, cabs drive in and out of the large garden gates, and students with heavy books intermingle with the crowd. The hospital is heir to both Ottoman surgery and European medicine. Most physicians there speak proudly of the influence of French and German schools of medicine[25] and how surgery, which was believed to be the highest medical practice of all, was first practiced in Turkey in these buildings.

The anatomy lab was the largest of its kind in Turkey and it distributed cadavers to the entire nation. As I walked in, the smell of preservatives mixed with white fluorescent lights and the odor of chemicals evaporating off the skin of the dead. The refreshing views of the Bosporus were far away now, yet so near. This was neither paradise nor its other side.

The large basement level occupied by the lab included one very large room in which each professor had a desk; another room in which the director had his own office, and other rooms for nurses and assistants. All appeared quite messy, filled with dilapidated furniture, shelves of outdated encyclopedias, and stacks of dusty papers. Separated from the offices, occupying the other half of the floor, was a large dissection room with eight tables. Until recently, dead bodies had been stored in a pool of formalin in the big room next door. By the time I saw the lab, the pool of the dead had been replaced by about a dozen freezers, each with three berths for three cadavers.

The pool of the dead was gone, but its image was still vivid in my mind. I recalled a conversation I had had with one of the brain surgeons from the mental hospital. "It is a shame," he said, "a shame for the medical community to have a swimming pool in which the bodies of the mentally ill are dumped." These were patients abandoned to a life of exile in the mental hospital. For many years they had lived in a half-shocked, half-drugged condition, enduring with only a single set of clothing and a meager diet until their lives came to an end. And then they were thrown into a common pool in the basement of a hospital, a place that no one could know about. As I was in the dissecting room looking around, I recalled Osman's impressions, and began imagining the pool of the dead behind the door where it used to be.

> It is a dark and cold place. The pool is a large swimming pool with blue tiles. It is filled with this very heavy-smelling chemical substance that gets into your clothes and skin if you stay there too long. And then when you look at the pool, you see corpses just floating in there. It is like a scene from a horror movie, or a tragedy. Few people know about this place. Even though most of the doctors know that they learn dissection on the corpses of the mental patients, they are not supposed to know how these bodies are preserved in the pool of the dead. It took me a long time to get permission to see it. I heard about it when I was there in the anatomy lab looking for a brain for dissection. After all those years they finally replaced the pool with normal preservation cabinets. But for decades anatomists have been working next to this pool. To me it was hard to believe. It was a dramatic change in my life; seeing it, I felt I crossed the line.

In a country where dying marked the line that separated the normal from the taboo, that separated the *jann* from the lifeless, and that prevented any exchange with the dead, it was difficult for doctors to accept seeing dead bodies treated like this. Osman's personal experience—his changed feelings upon seeing so many bodies collected in a common pool—testified to the power of death and the value of the dead body in Turkey. To Osman death was something that gave meaning to ideals and to the practice of one's vocation. In his time off from his job at the mental hospital, he also took care of patients sent to him by the Human Rights Foundation in Istanbul; most of these were political prisoners who had been on hunger strikes, people who had risked their lives for their political ideals. He had been a political prisoner himself after the putsch of 1980. Back then, he was ready to fight and die for his ideals, like many others, to save Turkey from inequalities and oppression. Dying at the mental hospital and being delivered to the anatomy lab meant exclusion from ideals, exclusion from politics, and exclusion from society. The miserable conditions of life and death in the mental hospital, the anatomy lab, and such modern cemeteries as the pool of the dead were signs that the medical community was unable to fulfill its commitment to serving people. It was as if the lives of these mentally ill people had no value. Their bodies were treated like objects, and this was not what humans deserved. This was the threshold for Osman. No matter how a person lived or died, a dead body should not be treated like any common object.

Tolstoy's well-known aphorism, "It is not how one lives, but how one dies that gives meaning to one's life," resonated for Osman and his generation of Turkish physicians, who were influenced by Russian romanticism and German idealism. In terms of this romantic idealism, a desire to live in a world of equality and justice, and his own ideas of revolution and social reform, Osman felt marginalized by the practices of his vocation. He felt the value he attached to life was also being marginalized.

Dr. Feridun Vural, the head of the anatomy lab at Cerrahpaşa University Hospital, was similarly upset about the conditions in which anatomy was taught: using the dead bodies of the most vulnerable, and until recently not even preserving them properly. Dr. Mehmet, an assistant anatomist, shared Vural's views. Anatomists' salaries were very low. They could not talk to anyone outside the hospital about the work they did, and they were looked down upon within the medical community as the "poor" "unskilled" doctors who could never achieve anything more than working on the bodies of the dead.[26]

Understanding anatomists' and surgeons' discomfort about the bodies they used for dissection depends on understanding the dual meaning death holds for them: on the one hand is the cultural understanding of death; on the other hand is the scientific and medical value of the dead bodies of the mentally ill in Turkey. These doctors were confronted by the conditions of their own vocation, conditions that they could neither avoid nor change because the epistemology of modern medicine in which they were immersed was built upon the physical unmaking of the human body. It was "an *impossible* endeavor in a country like Turkey," one of them said, complaining about the culture from which doctors could not separate their practice. The miserable circumstances of dissection mirrored for a moment the failures in the medical venture.

I was often moved as I listened to anatomists, nurses, and assistants confront their helplessness and saw the taboos they struggled with, how they questioned life and death, poverty and misery in Turkey. They had a deep personal engagement with their society on a daily basis as they practiced medicine, dissecting dead bodies, teaching students, and trying not to be seen as simply brutal and heartless for cutting apart the dead bodies of the abandoned and mentally ill. They believed that there was hostility toward their profession: they had the lowest funding and the least respectability among all other spheres of medicine. Part of the reason was the nature of their work involving dead bodies. The main reason for their marginalization, however, was the financial cul-de-sac in which they found themselves. Anatomy was the one field in medicine where there were no prospects for professional or financial advancement.[27] It was the only field that was almost entirely oriented toward education and had no commercial dimension. This affected everything from anatomists' research to the way they had set up their labs and stored and preserved cadavers. "Our misfortune is doing science [bilim] in a medical establishment where applications and technology are supposed to lead toward material and individual success," Dr. Mehmed told me. Anatomists could not earn a decent enough salary or gain control over enough funds for their labs to secure a good reputation, and as a result, they could not gain sufficient political power within hospital and university administrations to improve their facilities. After thirty-three years of struggle with the university, Dr. Vural at last managed to have the anatomy lab facilities and office spaces upgraded—not because the medical system started valuing basic science more, but because the new president had made him a promise long ago. At last the pool of the dead was replaced with freezers; anatomists were given larger office spaces and dissection rooms.

From one side, the power of death, stemming from the taboos that surround it, loomed over the anatomists. From the other, a general disinterest toward science and research structured the culture of anatomy. The modern space of death devalued scientific research and degraded the respectability of the vocation, and these effects were exacerbated by market pressures on medical practice. It was unclear which marginalized anatomy more: death, poverty, or lack of confidence in anatomy's scientific value.

BEYOND THE MIRROR

My field experiences in the spaces of death led me to believe that the dead body was believed to start a new kind of life in the cemetery. The cadaver, however, had a different destiny. It started a new kind of life in the anatomy lab. The transformation of a dead body into a cadaver was a profound experience for anatomists, one that shaped their vocation and the human condition in the depths of medical practice.

The invention of the cadaver was a bureaucratic procedure to begin with. To comply with legal procedures and get consent for dissection, Vural would send a letter to the family of the deceased informing them of the death and the location of the body; he also explained that the body would be used for medical research in the anatomy lab if the family did not claim it. In more than thirty years in the anatomy lab, Vural had seen families come to the lab upon receiving these letters in order to have their relatives' dead bodies fished out of the pool of the dead—families who might not have seen their relatives for decades, who had abandoned them in the mental hospital. Regardless of how little these people cared about their family members' welfare in the mental hospital, *after death* they would start treating them like normal people. There was an urgency to bury the dead; family members would not give consent for dissection.

When Vural met with the family members, he would tell them that a cadaver was something special. It was serving a holy purpose for a brief period of time; it was serving society by serving medical education. This was a sort of labor, he told them, and it was not an infinite task. After being used for anatomical research, the cadaver would be buried like any other body. To be more persuasive, he would emphasize that this was merely a "transitional phase" (*geçiçi bir dönem*), or sometimes he would call it "a transitional phase in service of humanity." He wanted the families to have a good feeling about the destiny of the bodies, that these bodies could at last be functional in society, even if only for a brief period of time.

With this invention of a transitional public service phase between death and burial—the dead body becoming a cadaver and the lab becoming a liminal space like the cemetery but not really a place of rest—anatomy was undoing the common-sense understandings of the life cycle. The new transitional phase was between death and burial; it was a new kind of existence, destabilizing the arrangement of cosmological space and the value of the cemetery. Despite its virtues, Vural's "transitional phase" did not convince the families. They resisted the invention of this new time and new life for the dead body and refused to donate.

The truth was that the transitional phase was an ambiguous mode of existence in the context of the traditional Turkish Sunni Muslim understanding of time as well as the metaphysical and cosmological construction of spatial existence. This spatialization was central to religious doctrine and a daily religious practice—Friday prayers were full of references to the cycles

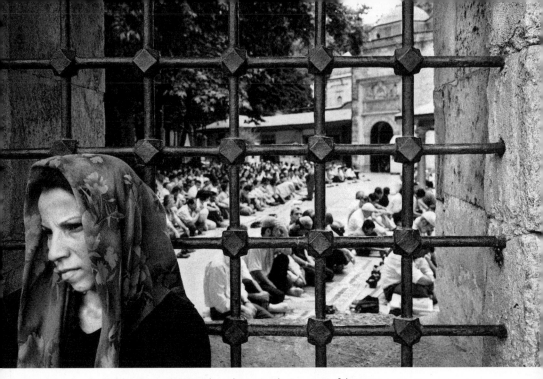

8. "Friday Prayer at Eyüp" by Laleper Aytek. Courtesy of the artist.

of life and the meaning of moral acts in this world.[28] The imam of Eyüb Sultan, for instance, referred to the afterlife as a starting point, as the true reality giving meaning and legitimate form to action in this world. "We have two lives: one in this world, a life of trials, and another life in the afterlife as immortal beings. The existence of heaven and hell in the afterlife gives meaning to our lives in this world," he told the crowds of men inside the mosque and the women praying outside during a Friday prayer. Afterlife was a part of the knowledge of the self; the crowd of worshippers nodded in agreement as the imam spoke.

In the sequence of life, death, and immortality, ways of being were temporally arranged as forms of existence in space—from this world to the mosque, to the cemetery, and then to resurrection and the afterlife—of which time was merely a derivative. This was in marked contrast to the scientific conception of biological life and modernity, however, in which change was understood on the basis of the passage of time and labor. The "transitional phase" was a human intervention in this divine order.[29] Anatomists had no other means to convince the families to consent but to invent a new time frame so that the cadaver's brief life in the laboratory made sense, so that it could be internalized as a part of the Muslim cosmology. But the invention of the transitional phase seemed to disrupt the traditional schema rather than fitting into it. The anatomy lab was not just another spatial phase, stable and familiar. The activity of dissection threatened to divest the human being of its self-same personhood, to transform it into a commodity, an object, and to instrumentalize it for purposes other than the passage of the soul through cosmological space. The transitional phase not only physically altered the body but in effect reduced it to a commodity by measuring its value according to worldly time as labor. Although its virtues failed to achieve its goal of persuading families to donate their relatives' bodies, it did alter the way anatomists viewed the dead body: the cadavers came to be animated by these notions of the time of the transitional phase and the labor of serving medical education.

One of the things that struck me most as I watched dissection was how physicians treated and spoke about the cadavers. During dissection, these bodies were not treated as dead, but almost like living bodies on an operating table by virtue of their status serving society. This imaginary *jann* made the bodies seem as if they were doing an *insani* (humane) thing for society after their death. Anatomists were careful and quiet as they worked on bodies because of their "respect for the humane qualities of the cadaver." They were very conscious of dissection's interference with the cosmology of life and death as it created a new existence for the dead. Instead of lying in the earth, the dead bodies were lying on hard tables in cold, damp laboratory rooms. Instead of being alone, decaying into the earth, they were being artificially preserved, turning strange colors and taking on a sharp chemical smell. The new life of the dead haunted the anatomists much more than it did the families of the deceased. It imprisoned them in their own construction of time. Anatomists took the body from the realm of death and relocated it in the realm of the living. In this new time the body became sort of alive—a life-less object—as it performed its service with its imaginary *jann*. By placing the dead body in the realm of the living, anatomists felt they were working on a "respectable human," as they worded it.

One day, I was in the dissection room, looking around and waiting for Dr. Ali, the lab assistant, to prepare his tools for dissection. The room was cold and damp. It contained a few sinks and eight dissection tables. A few cadavers were laid out, covered with wet green cloths that prevented their flesh from drying out. One of the mirrors mounted on the wall above the sinks caught my attention. It was covered in large, dark, shadowy stains. It looked as if something had spoiled the image from the outside. Other mirrors were in the same condition. As I began to examine them more closely I heard Ali say, "It is nothing, really." I had not been planning on asking him about it. But seeing that I did not respond, he continued, "These are all new mirrors. The carpenter used the wrong glue and it got onto the surface of the mirror, so now all our mirrors in this room are stained. It is nothing, just the silicone glue . . . really, it is nothing." When I looked at the mirror, I could see Mehmed's body over my shoulder. Yet a dark shadow on the surface of the mirror stood between his body and its reflection, spoiling his image. At that moment, with Ali's repetitive explanation, it seemed as if Mehmed's soul was trapped somewhere on the mirror's surface. His image was not where it was supposed to be, in the reflected depth beyond the mirror.

His mirror image was spoiled.[30] Had Ali not told me over and over again that the stains were silicon and nothing more, it would not even have occurred to me that some metaphysical cause lay behind the spoiled mirror image. In the dissection lab, a space that until recently had had the pool of the dead right next to it, a normal mirror image would be a stabilizing influence. For this reason, it seemed, the spoiled mirror image was a great embarrassment to Ali. He continued complaining about the carpenter and the poor quality of the construction, and he repeated the story each time we were in the dissection room.

As Ali demonstrated the dissection procedure on Mehmed's body, he was very caring and tender. He spoke continuously about the cadaver—his age, the state of his body—and said that it was important to be gentle with it and try not to damage it so that it would not feel mistreated while performing its service to society. Mehmed was neither dead nor alive on that table. As such, Ali was making associations with the traditional Turkish construction of the body-soul and its displacement in the lab during dissection. It was not life as common sense ruled that flowed through Mehmed's veins as he lay on the dissection table. But his service, his labor during the transitional phase of his being, animated him. In Ali's hands, the dead Mehmed became an uncanny being, more alive than dead, yet even more enslaved than he was in life. The anatomist was inventing an identity for him, one that went beyond his former life at the asylum and the oppressed existence that preceded it. While the mirror ushered the cadaver back into worldly life, at the same time it reflected the continuum of everyday violence in which the scientific setting of the lab was located. It was thus, on the shoulders of the disadvantaged, that anatomy operated as an exploration of the body and a science of culture.

Ali, viewing a dead body, felt the need to animate it, to bring it back to life in order to make it a part of his practice. However, bringing the dead back to life also caused a backlash in spite of the body's decontextualization and its reduction from a human being to a cadaver—to an object. Vural had told me a short anecdote, which I could not forget. One night when he was a young assistant, he was dissecting in the middle of the night and had not realized how the time had passed and the lab had emptied. He was still in the dissection room, cutting open the skull of a cadaver with a saw to dissect the brain. Suddenly, for some reason, he stopped and looked at the cadaver. Its eyes were open and they stared at him as he tried to get into the brain. "I froze," he said. "I do not know how it happened, but all of a sudden I realized I was all alone in the middle of the night cutting into the skull of a dead human being. What was I doing there in the middle of the night? I got so scared. I threw the saw onto the floor, packed all my stuff, and ran away. Since then I have never worked there alone at night."

Knowing that the cadavers came from a life of institutionalization in the mental hospital, the anatomists had to find ways to humanize the dead bodies so as to protect themselves from projections of violence. The institution of which they were a part had participated in the construction of the concept of insanity, created a physical space for its treatment, and made the dissection of these bodies a prerequisite for its own scientific advancement. This vicious circle, which started with the creation of the insane and ended with the study of their flesh, unfolded in isolated spaces far from public view, hidden behind high walls and in the basements of hospitals. All of it was beyond the normalcy of events that constituted the human. For anatomists, anxiety and vocational failure mixed with the effort required to make dead bodies into objects of study. Trauma took hold of their vocation; time and space froze, chaining the unclaimed souls of the mentally ill and the anatomists alike. In this parallel universe of the biopolis, neither biological change nor the possibility of liberation was allowed. The other side of the *unknowable* captured the emptied bodies of these people whose escape, whose labor, and whose renaming could not be completed.

DISSECTION AND DISENCHANTMENT

The first Turkish anatomy atlas, *Hamse-i Şânîzâde*, was published by the physician Şânîzâde in 1820. It was a time shortly before the Tanzimat, the Ottoman reformation of 1839–76. The first printing press in the Muslim world had been introduced one hundred years earlier by İbrahim Müteferrika, but no more than sixty books had been published throughout the eighteenth century in the Ottoman Empire.[31] The first of *Hamse's* five volumes on anatomy was titled *The Mirror of the Body Inside the Anatomy of Human Organs (Mirâtü'l-Ebdân fi Tesrih-i Âzâü'l-İnsân)*.[32] Şânîzâde's introduction to *The Mirror of the Body* stressed the importance of medicine in the age of reformation and enlightenment: "Medicine and anatomy are natural sciences and the core of human knowledge. These sciences are complex; their subject matter involves the body and religion. They are the disciplines that see the truth, and as such they have been praised by many intelligent and rational people as the most valuable and respectable fields of study since ancient times. Their research not only includes the human kind . . . but all creatures that believe in and are created by God."[33]

When *Hamse* was published, Şânîzâde presented a copy of the finished work to the Sultan, Mahmud II. The sultan then sent an elegantly prepared copy to the French embassy, which caught the attention of the Orientalist Bianchi, who would later write on the pioneering nature of Şânîzâde's work and the Ottomans' advanced knowledge.[34] The 1820s had seen increased political interest by the French in the East, while the Ottomans began feeling threatened by French military domination in the Mediterranean. The sultan's gift of the book *Hamse* may have been intended to demonstrate to the French that the Ottomans were their civilizational equals, as they too valued science, rational thinking, and disenchantment.

For Şânîzâde, the mirroring as a reflection of the inside of the body was a means of enlightenment. It was about exteriorizing and illuminating; it was a statement of liberation. In a similar fashion, the struggle of anatomists for a legitimate place within the medical community was reflected in the ways they related to contemporary Turkish literature. Like the enlightenment reflected in the making of art and literature, they viewed dissection as analogous to traditional philosophies of illumination.[35] Science, in this sense, was viewed as an outlet of light, liberation, and consciousness.

On a few occasions while I conversed with the assistant anatomists in their lab, they invoked Turkish poetry in a way that served not only as a common cultural referent, but illuminated for a moment their feelings of marginalization. The poet the anatomists invoked was Küçük İskender, a leading figure in the literature and gay politics of the 1990s. Küçük İskender started publishing his poems in the late 1980s. His poems described the inner secrets of the body and the experience of pain and violence in private life. He wrote about nudity, sex, and death. He undid the privacy of the person by invoking images of blood and internal organs. By speaking of the biological body, he spoke of the most intimate feelings. By transgressing cultural taboos, he liberated language, thought, and the place of sexuality in social life.

> Oysa toprak bize daima ihanet etti
> Gövdemizi ihmal etti
> Gövdemizi yemek icin gövdemizi besledi
> Gövde, katlandı. Sık sık akineton yuttu.
> Gövde gösterilmedi. Işıkla soğutuldu saklandı.

> Yet the earth had actually betrayed us
> It neglected our bodies
> It fed our bodies to eat our bodies
> The body endured. By swallowing drugs [akineton].
> The body was not displayed. It was frozen by light. It was kept
> [preserved].[36]

While in the Muslim tradition nudity was a taboo, bodily integrity and modesty were essential for a dignified life.[37] Contemporary Turkish popular culture had different techniques of dealing with the body. Its integrity if not its nudity was viewed as an integral part of personhood. By dissecting the nude body, and then not even putting it back together as surgeons would, Turkish anatomists were violating its integrity. Not surprisingly, the anatomists identified with Küçük İskender's work. Anatomists recognized that people lived with taboos against touching the body, speaking about it, and seeing its exposed parts. This was even true of many anatomists themselves—even among them there was a low rate of cadaver donation. According to a recent study on anatomists' attitudes toward cadaver donation, only around 15 percent of them were willing to donate, whereas approximately 65 percent were against it. Among the many reasons, they cited the reluctance to be dissected by a colleague, fear of hurting their "family members' feelings," "general psychological" reasons, and anxiety about the "disrespectful treatment of the cadaver." A few anatomists had strong "religious drives" that prevented them from donating their bodies.[38] Their reactions paralleled those in other Middle Eastern countries.[39] Most of the anatomists believed that the best solution would be to increase the supply of unclaimed bodies from hospitals because it was impossible to convince the public of the value of organ and cadaver donation.

The internal body was a private realm where the self resided: what was inside should remain inside. The way the anatomists penetrated the boundary of the skin and the depths of the flesh to view organs and internal parts of the body was an unusual thing, a transgressive practice in which they engaged in spite of the culture beyond the doors of the lab. They practiced a borderline vocation, turning bodies inside out, as the poet Küçük İskender did in his poetry. The way he redefined words and brought them back to their physical actuality was analogous to the way anatomists challenged themselves to become disenchanted practitioners amid the cultural taboos surrounding nudity and bodily integrity. Like the poet did in words, the anatomists were trying to bring things out into the open for rediscovery.

> Onlar İ.O. öldüler
> Bir açıklama bahanesi ile
> Renksiz kokusuz ve tensiz kadavra.
> Miadi dolmuş bir beden bu. çürük. kirli.
> Pasaklı. kullanılmış. satılmış.

> They died in BC.
> Excusing itself with an explanation
> Colorless odorless and skinless cadaver.
> A body long overdue. rotten. dirty.
> Filthy. abused. sold.[40]

Küçük İskender's poems used body parts, organs, and bodily fluids as metaphors to speak of social life. He depicted the traditional understanding of the body, the earth, death, decay, and what was to come after as the opiate of Turkish cosmology. In his bodies there was no beauty but ugliness, no future but mortality—there was neither dignity nor integrity. He told of a truth embodied in death and manifested in a cadaver—an object—not an exotic or sacred dead body. Things we have learned to romanticize and exoticize about life were absent even in his verses on love. His work was like that of a psychoanalyst, bringing the inside of things out to the world, disenchanting the self by speaking of its parts. These metaphors worked well in words, verses, poems of modernity. Anatomists' attachment to Küçük İskender's poetry was symptomatic; it illustrated their marginalization in their own society for dissecting the body, bringing the secrets of the body out to the external world. Disenchantment and dissection were analogous terms for the anatomists, who worked on the bodies of the abandoned, who could not speak much about their vocation outside the lab doors, and who had to invent an artificial intervention in the life cycle—the transitional phase—in order to be able to pursue their practice. One anatomist believed they were artists of the body.

BURIAL

These anatomists fought battles in invisible corners of modern institutions, far from everyday life, further away from people's attachment to traditions. Vural thought that Muslim traditions and values, deeply rooted in the Turkish people's mindset, were the root cause of the extremely low donations of cadavers to anatomy—only six or seven bodies throughout all his professional life. In spite of all of the efforts at modernization, the spirit of religion ultimately determined the value of all things. Economic sensibilities were also mixed in. People had feelings of ownership and stewardship toward the dead body just like those they held toward their homes and land: they felt responsible for the care of these things. Vural believed that dead bodies in Turkey were treated as though they were more valuable than the living. Other anatomists in the department agreed with him: "Turkish people would leave a person, abandon him, never take care of him when he is alive; but when [he] is dead, the body all of a sudden becomes valuable. No one wants the dead body to be touched or to be thrown away like an ordinary object."

Vural thought possessiveness was the main drive for this kind of subject-property relationship. People felt obliged toward their dead, began viewing their relatives' dead bodies as their own, as objects to which they became heir. Even if a person had left a letter donating his or her body for dissection, the family often felt uncomfortable taking responsibility for executing this decision for this reason. Moreover, physicians thought, like land or a house, Turkish people wanted to own, not rent, when it came to the body. They gave me an example from the urban landscape of Istanbul. The poorest would build one-story houses in a slum and leave an iron rebar frame above the building so that they could build a second floor when they had more income; everyone wanted to own space. "They [families] want to say 'it's mine,'" Vural told me, "'I own this.'" When a family member died, the heirs owned the dead body along with the other properties of the inheritance. From the time of death to the time of burial, the body was theirs. That was why there was an urgency to bury the dead body, Vural had observed all these years.

Traditionally before any inheritance can be distributed among family members, the deceased must be buried. The funeral and the burial fulfilled the last obligations to the deceased. The immediate burial separated the body from the properties it was attached to in life, which now, after death, would become objects of inheritance. In principle, *fıkıh* books (Islamic law) specified in detail the structure of burial rites in order to stabilize this liminal sphere of economic transaction. The soul had to retreat to its place in the grave to be detached from its worldly property. After the funeral was over, the second important obligation to the deceased would be paying any remaining debts from the inheritance money. Once these tasks were completed, family members would try to fulfill the dead person's will, if there was one. The final stage of inheritance rites was the subsequent distribution of property.[41] The "transitional phase" complicated matters.

Scholars of Islamic law suggested that recent medical technologies have changed the tradition: one could no longer posit absolute definitions of personhood and bodily integrity; one could not expect medicine to be held back because of taboo and rigid categories of bodily propriety. Autopsy, dissection, and organ transplantation were all fields that challenged the categories whose aim was to protect the dignity and integrity of the body. The rights of the person were viewed as a primary principle of social life.[42] As such, violating the dead or the living body was viewed as violating personhood. The issue of *emanet*, the borrowed nature of the body, complicated matters. The body was the person's *responsibility* in life. But it was also the person's *possibility*: with the body one could live, breathe, exchange, be social—in short exist. All these vanished for the body in death. Dead, one was no longer a person.

In Islamic cosmology, there were two distinct categories that constituted personhood. The category *insan*, the human, was the universal to which all humans belonged regardless of their mental health, color, sex, or maturity; it was the theological equivalent to the scientific category *Homo sapiens*. "All were born human"; all souls that reside in human bodies were human.[43] The *insan* constituted the nominal subject of public law, an entity inherently endowed with the capacity to participate in social life. Personhood (*şahsiyet*), however, was the superior category of the two and was determined by means of *mahremiyet* (private law). Not all humans were regarded as full or rational *persons*. To participate in legal-communal life, one had to have *akıl*, or reason, and be past the age of legal adulthood, in republican Turkey, eighteen. This even used to apply to suicides in the past: to be ritually buried as a full Muslim person, one should not have committed suicide.[44]

Islamic law regarding medicine and the body of the person was negotiated within the category of the material rights of the body and was concerned with the protection of a person's privacy in this worldly life. To this end, material rights were the rights over the body, and the right to privacy (*mahremiyet*) was the right of the soul (*ruh*). Besides these, personhood also permitted access to economic life. The rights of the person (*şahsiyet hakları*) were different from the rights of the *human* in this value system, and less value was attached to the universal category of the human. Beyond the universal category *insan* (human) and the legal socioeconomic category *şahsiyet* (person) remained the outcasts, the non-persons like the mentally ill and the homeless whose bodies could remain unclaimed after their deaths. In the classical Greek tradition this category was called *zoë*, the life inherent in all beings but not distinct to humans. Because of being in a subhuman category the mentally ill, the homeless, and other people of exclusion whose bodies go unclaimed are legally considered as less than persons and analogously viewed as less human, and in today's emerging economies their dead bodies could be made life-less.

The Qur'an and the collected *hadis* (hadith) of Muhammed called the *sünnet* (Sunnah)—the two main sources laying out the moral and legal principles of Muslim daily life[45]—contain verses and sayings that seem to ban violations to the living body and to the graves of dead persons.

However, a practice such as autopsy insofar as it helps reveal the truth cannot be regarded as a violation. This falls under the general principle that to prevent a larger crime, a minor violation may be permitted and may even be imperative.[46] While this was the general approach to dissection and autopsy in Turkey, the Ministry of Justice in Saudi Arabia, to which Turkish Muslim scholars of the Sunni tradition sometimes turned, has issued stricter views on medical research on cadavers. It has allowed corpses to be used as evidence in solving crimes or for research on infectious diseases, but it has also concluded that in spite of Islam's respect for science and education, anatomical dissection for medical training should be limited to the bodies of executed criminals. The cadaver is as valuable as the living body, if not in some ways more so, and for this reason it is difficult to reincorporate it into the world of education without raising questions about the maintenance of bodily integrity. Since those who received the death penalty were regarded as non-persons, their dead bodies could be pushed to the outskirts of the moral and economic system. In this sense, their place in anatomy resembled that of the mentally ill elsewhere. These could be treated as if they had no personhood. The anatomists were caught in the ambiguous legal-theological language they wished to interpret and appropriate in order to be able to dissect these bodies, yet at the same time they had to silence the problems that arose between the dead and themselves.

RITES OF DIFFUSION

To me, the anatomists' unease posed two questions about life and death: What were the techniques and contextualizing discourses that made the "human," the "person," or the "non-person" distinct from an animal and close to an object? And how did physicians handle medical practices, invent rituals, and view their place in society through these techniques and discourses in the emerging biopolis?

Arnold van Gennep, in his research on the changes in status performed in burial and reburial and other rituals, famously theorized such practices as *rites of passage* consisting of three stages: *separation, transition* or *liminality,* and *incorporation.*[47] The rites of passage were conducted for the common human being to incorporate into different cycles of existence through certain rituals.

The passage of the dead in the anatomy lab, however, was incomplete. In spaces of death like the dissection room, speechless communities resided[48]—somewhat like Turner's communitas, or perhaps more like Taussig's colonial subjects—dead but alive, invisible but present. I thought of these silent presences in terms of metaphors of social life that challenged dissection and its practitioners from within, altering the vision of the anatomist as they imagined being absorbed by the eye of the cadaver. I asked further: Was it proper to perform work on the body of a silenced human being? What kind of knowledge would be gained through its body? How would the transitions of a marginal person like Mehmed be accomplished if the collective did not desire to incorporate or recognize these transitions?

Anatomists had invented a discourse of labor that attributed respect, dignity, and integrity to the dead body. With it they hoped to restore a non-person to personhood. Yet it almost seemed as if this ritual process accomplished the inverse process: the closer anatomists came to the cadaver, the more they internalized it. The more they internalized it, the more they absorbed its tainted meaning—not the meaning implied in its non-person human condition, but rather its history of isolation and oppression. An uncanny feeling, as Vural spoke of in many occasions, surfaced. This uncanny feeling marked their unconscious language. Freud had said that "the uncanny was what one called everything that was meant to remain secret and hidden and has come into the open."[49] Tracing the semantics of the word *heimlich*, meaning familiar, he suggests that its antonym, *unheimlich*, or "uncanny," represented the revelation of the repressed, the mysterious, and the unwanted. The uncanny signified a kind of relation. The anatomists' relationship with the cadaver embodied this form. It was conducted as a reburial rite that had the respectable restoration of the cadaver and the science of anatomy as its desired goal. As the cadaver decayed and its skin became a dirty brown color, it reached out to the material world. With dissection, the *unknown* was made *known*. Through tainted mirrors and eyes frozen open, the secrets of the mental hospital, the secrets of the naked body, the secrets of insanity had been revealed. These secrets had become the personal knowledge of the anatomists.

As anatomists entered the transitional phase with the cadaver, they invented a discourse that fulfilled their wishes and made the cadaver more human. The anatomists sought, by attributing qualities of labor and respectability to the cadaver, to be able to perform dissection on the body of a "legitimate" person. The space of death of the lab became a microcosm of their rite of passage.

High-tech medicine had invented a rite of passage, or what I call a *rite of diffusion*, in which the body was internalized as consisting of spare parts for other bodies or as raw material to enrich scientific practice in the biopolis's economy of the human body and emotions. The rite of diffusion was a new rite of passage intended to restore the memory of the deceased but also to use its dead body for the corpus of knowledge and reapportion parts for the social corpus. How could the unclaimed bodies of the mentally ill be restored to a condition that was functional yet still humane? The pool of the dead, in which the corpses swam side by side, had already exaggerated the uncanny condition of the cadaver, which was penetrated and preserved by the formaldehyde instead of being ritually washed in the mosque and left to decay in the earth. The formaldehyde chemically purified the body, like the radiation or demineralization techniques in allografts, killing its texture; what already was a non-person became petrified while its suppressed memories materialized in its new form. But to the naked eye the preserved body was anything but pure, for the naked eye can see nearer to the truth than any other device. Preservation and dissection could not cleanse and purify the violence inflicted by social life. On the contrary, the anatomists' practice revealed this violence. Unable to separate themselves from the cadaver during this person-to-non-person relationship, the anatomists, I thought, identified with it more intensely the deeper they cut into the cadaver. The identification process projected itself onto the discourse of the respectable cadaver, as the anatomists began inhabiting the uncanny.

Anatomy's rite of diffusion was traumatic. The cadaver was internalized without purification: no discourse, not even that of the transitional phase, was sufficient; no word, not even "respectability," could save it; no burial could make it a full person. The bodies of the mentally ill were marginalized excluded bodies unlike the assimilated allografts imported in plastic bags from foreign lands. The *kadavra* could not become inert within the epistemics of anatomy as exercised in Turkey. While orthopedic surgeons used allografts with ease and without much reflection, anatomists confronted exclusion. And in time, the secrets of everyday violence became the chains of medical education, solidified in the corpses of the unclaimed. Many remembered their anatomy education in conjunction with the coup, street fights, zones of abandonment, and other maladies and tensions of political life for this reason.

Anatomy's aim was not to reveal secrets of social life but to illuminate the mechanisms of the Cartesian body—the enlightenment Şânîzâde had once hoped for. The uncanny demonstrated the impossibility of maintaining an artificial life cycle for the dead body in the realm of the living, the impossibility of a science of the dissected unclaimed body, and the power of the spaces of death in this world. Spaces of death—physical, metaphysical, and a variety of parallel worlds between the two—were all spaces of liminality.[50] Relying on socially disadvantaged groups and traditional theological categories, physicians practiced medicine in these worlds, transgressing and transforming their practices through the diffused bodies of their subjects. The liminal condition affected their practice through identification and projection mechanisms while they tried to maintain normalcy, regularity, and propriety in practice.

Likewise, commodification of the dead body affected biomedicine and its changing epistemology. Physicians felt chained in a set of epistemic circumstances from which they wanted to be liberated while still being able to practice medicine and utilize technology. The bioscientific rite of passage—the rites of diffusion—took place in these processes of knowledge production within the biopolis. It took place in spaces of exclusion that revealed repressed social mechanisms during the anatomist's individual journey through the liminal condition. It was a drama of techniques and contextualizing discourses. It was a collectively suppressed human condition that changed institutional and social mechanisms. Transplant surgeons learned dissection in the same labs and improved their skills by working on living bodies in time. They had learned medicine, dissection, and surgery, all of which were rooted in such rites of diffusion to begin with.

A trauma was inflicted by the unclaimed body's use as an object of knowledge in the dissection room. The rite of diffusion was a way for anatomists to think about their unease, to rationalize their use of a body, to accord it a kind of personhood. Transplant surgeons would utilize the same social technique to invent the brain-dead donor to be able to transplant from the *kadavra*.

REBURIAL

> Whoever kills a soul unless it be for manslaughter or for corruption on the earth, as if he killed all humanity. Whoever keeps him alive, as if he kept alive all the humanity.
>
> —QUR'AN 5:32

Similar to the efforts of anatomists who were trying to invent the "respectable" cadaver from the mentally ill, transplant surgeons in search of a stable pool of cadaveric donors in Turkey would mobilize the media and the state institutions to justify a small yet stable donor pool for transplants.[51] They had to invent a life-less body whose reburial could be completed. This was how I heard of Ebru Esler, twenty-one, and her husband, Murat, twenty-four, a couple newly married, and living and working in Istanbul. Reminiscent of David Lynch's films, Ebru had killed her husband and then attempted to commit suicide. The police had arrived on the scene to find her still alive. After six hours of struggle to keep her alive in a nearby hospital, at midnight the doctors told her parents that they were unable to save her life, that she was brain dead.[52] The mother had then given consent for organ donation. The body was transported to Istanbul University Hospital and delivered to Dr. Eldegez's transplant team for organ harvesting.

The next day, the Turkish public awoke to a media campaign announcing the increasing number of dialysis patients throughout the nation, some twenty thousand at that time, and decrying the suffering they endured. In interviews doctors spoke about the long waiting lists for organs and the virtues of organ donation. The Minister of Health declared Ebru a heroine: in spite of having killed her husband, she had saved six people's lives. With the story becoming headlines in papers, doctors called on everyone to fill out organ donation cards as a legacy to their loved ones.[53] The media campaign was provocative; it mobilized hundreds of people, increasing the amount of signed organ donation cards by four times.[54] The media professionals, who had recently lost one of their colleagues for lack of a cadaveric liver, took up the case and turned it into a legend.[55] In a departure from their prior tendency always to bring up the so-called organ mafia in every transplantation story, this time the reporting was supportive, and Eldegez publicly expressed his gratitude.[56]

In the days and months to come, the media started focusing on the lives and stories of the patients who were saved by Ebru's organs. Her heart found a place in a man in Istanbul, her liver was flown to İzmir to another man, and one of her kidneys was given to a mother in Istanbul.[57] A couple of months later, the patient who had received Ebru's liver met with four other patients who had received organs from cadavers that had been donated after Ebru's suicide. They met at a hospital in İzmir and thanked the donors in prayers. "May those who have given us life rest in peace, in light [*nur içinde yatsınlar*]," they said. "We are grateful to their families."[58]

Ebru's story became an archetype. Six months later, one of her friends was killed in a traffic accident while driving a truck without a license on a jammed highway in Istanbul. When she was delivered to the hospital, she, too, was diagnosed as brain dead. Her parents recalled their daughter's testimony: "If anything ever happens to me, please donate my organs like Ebru's." She had even told Ebru's mother of a recent dream that Ebru was calling her to join her. Reading this dream as a metaphysical sign from the beyond, a newspaper headline reported the donation story, underlining the dream's deeper message: "She knew she would die."[59]

The suicide, the homicide, and the traffic accident with a message had eased the grounds for cadaveric transplants. These ways of dying were inventing a cadaveric pool of donors for transplants like anatomy's *kadavra*, the mentally ill; it was allowing these young souls to become social again and to get internalized. A nephrologist had told me that around half of the organs harvested from cadavers in her unit came from the bodies of suicides in the beginning of the 2000s:

> It is a taboo and a sin to commit suicide in our religion. There is no intellectual, rational criterion for the place of suicide in social life—regarding the ethics of harvesting the organs of those who have committed suicide. . . . But which one is better? To encourage patients for living related donations when, as we all know, they exchange their kidneys for property anyway? We had such an experience here. . . . There was this girl who donated one of her kidneys to her father. The father had an organ rejection. Then he found another young woman from his village, and that woman sold him a kidney in exchange for an apartment. But then the daughter started having a deep depression from two losses: one was her own kidney and the other was the lack of appreciation of her altruistic donation. The living-to-living transplantations always involve some sort

of exchange in terms of a commodity. . . . The only case of transplantations where there is no exchange is among couples. They work very well, I must say. On the other hand, we have the cases of suicides in increasing rates every day. Their families have feelings of guilt. It is a sin to commit suicide; families do not know how to handle it. The Diyanet [Presidency of Religious Affairs] gave its consent for organ donation from brain-dead donors. . . . Even though these people have committed suicide, hence a sin, by organ donation they are given a chance to reverse the sin into a good deed by saving other people's lives.

By the act of donation, families were told, their loved ones would go to heaven in spite of the sin they had committed of taking their own lives, which did not belong to them to begin with. The Qur'anic sura Maide was invoked over and over again. The Diyanet's support of organ transplants was used as the fundamental ground by physicians who approached families for consent. It was as if harvesting a suicide's organs washed away the sin from the dead body, purified the person's life, restored his or her place back in the circle of the living.

The place of the dead among the living was changing. The media played an important role in the formation of this new place in the collective consciousness. It turned suicide into a positive end by which lives were being saved. It made organ harvesting from these bodies a desirable ethics. Transplants achieved a service to social life like no other field of medicine had ever done before: reforming the place of suicide in collective life. The brain-dead donor was finally invented as the soul of the suicide was restored in good memories, her past not erased but rewritten, her biography reinvented through the "reburial-donation."

A legend was born from tragedy and it took its place next to other mythic elements of the biopolis: the bone factory, the missing femurs and tibias of the deceased, and the American businessman's bag filled with bones. This one, unlike others, redeemed tragedy and turned it into an archetype. With it, suicide was technologically ritualized; a high-tech biopolis was inserted into the flow of life.[60] Technology such as this could transform the violence of everyday life to a common good. The impressions of Ebru's drama and its legendary qualities remained with me throughout my research. There, I could see suicide's changing face. It was one of the most profound elements of our collective life, its parameter, the measure of our human condition. When did this change start for Turkey, I asked myself. A donation, a media broadcast, a desirable death such as this could not come about from one day to the next. Anatomists had been struggling to find a supply of bodies for dissection for decades. "The respectable cadaver" and "the transitional phase" were phrases that disappeared into the void. The rites of diffusion were incomplete. How then could Eldegez's unit actually succeed in transforming the image of suicides for medical ends? What was the place of suicide in collective life in contemporary Turkey?

SUICIDE

No other way of dying isolated the *jann* from sociality like suicide. Not many people committed suicide in Turkey, as was the case throughout the Muslim world.[61] Suicide rates were much lower in predominantly Muslim countries, and Muslim minority communities also had lower suicide rates than other religious affiliations in other countries.[62] This negative correlation between suicide and Islam, however, did not necessarily indicate a positive outlook on life among Muslims. The public attitude toward suicide was complex. The effects of poverty, oppression, and isolation, the presence of the state and patriarchal structures, and changing human ideas about death and dying were all part of this complexity. In a new brave world, however, it was no longer sufficient to ask why people committed suicide. In my work, the more pressing question was how the state used the body of the suicide for biopolitical ends and for progress while transforming the place of death. Rites of passage did not have much room for reburials in anatomists' medical experience, but transplants could invent the reburial through Ebru's embodiment. The state's approach to suicide victims, together with that of the media, was a determining factor in the success of the Ebru legend.

Historically, in the early years of the Turkish republic, there had been an increase in suicides among both men and women. In a sociological study in the 1920s, it was even argued that the shock and alienation caused by the difficult transition of the reform years caused higher rates of suicide among women than among men and among Muslims than among Jewish or Christian minorities.[63] The suicide rates indicated the disproportionate effects of social reforms on the female body. Traditionally, the suicide rates among males were higher than females, whereas the number of attempted suicides among females was higher than among males. In the public history of suicides, there had been two exceptions to this ratio: the first one was in the early years of the republic, when the suicide rate among women rose but did not exceed the male rate; the second was in the province of Batman in southeastern Turkey in the 1990s and 2000s when female suicides exceeded males by 75 percent, giving Batman the second highest rate of suicide among women after China.[64] This was an extraordinary case.

While broadcasting the news of suicides, the media had followed very different approaches, censoring it in the early days of the republic and announcing it as a scandal as we approached the year 2000.[65] When the republic was young, the alarming suicides would have disturbed social solidarity at a time when it was most needed, and so the news had been censored. In the case of the suicides in Batman, the attention was overwhelming and significant for many reasons. It was actually about the changing relationship between the state and the subject. It was about Turkish modernization, the Kurdish question, the patriarchal structures of southeastern Turkey, and the value of the female body.[66] What in the 1920s and 1930s was a negative reflection, a fear of losing identity because of the rush to modernization, became a positive biopolitical discourse in the late 1990s and the early 2000s. Talk about suicide, donation, oppression, or salvation had begun marking the physical body upon the geographical space, and this talk could be mobilized for biopolitical ends.

In the early years of the republic, the regime change and radical reforms precipitated a sense of what Durkheim would call anomie or social alienation—a condition that gave rise to an increase in suicides. The legal force of Atatürk's reforms had penetrated so powerfully into daily life and in such a short period of time that basic ideas of family life were called into question.[67] In 1926 the new civil code was put into effect, changing some of the fundamental principles of family life. The new civil code banned polygamy, forcing men with polygynous households to choose one partner among many wives and at the same time giving women the right to divorce. In 1934 women were granted the right to vote and run for office. Shortly after the code was implemented, women began wearing modern dresses and abandoned the traditional veil.[68] Women's appearances, like their public rights and responsibilities, had changed in a short span of time; their place in social life had been altered dramatically and so had the way they viewed themselves and their marriages.[69] While women had been granted equality with their husbands in legal life, they had to carry these civil reforms sometimes as burdens into their private lives.

This was one of the main reasons for the increased rate of suicide among women in the early years of the reformation. Despite the decrease in suicides from 1929 to 1930, the numbers increased again in 1931. The increase forced the state to take measures. To prevent a public panic, a ban on newspaper reports of suicides was imposed that year. The ban had made the performance of burial rituals difficult. Until quite recently in modern-day Turkey, some imams in Anatolia would even refuse the traditional burial of suicides.[70] In the Hanefi school of Islamic law, suicide has been regarded as a greater sin than homicide. The body was an *emanet* from God, an object entrusted to the person for a lifetime; one could not violate the body's right to live.[71] This being a challenge in general for the families of the suicides, with the legal ban the families had to invent stories to explain the deaths of their loved ones so that they could announce the burial time and mosque in local newspapers. The publicity ban had reinforced the sin associated with suicide, but the public knew what was really going on when odd funeral announcements were printed in the papers.

> While the respectable so-and-so was hunting for butterflies, she fell out of the window. Her heavy head pulled her down.

> She died because the lines got around her neck while she was hanging the laundry.

> After she shot her lover, she was killed by a bullet from the rifle that had fallen on the ground.[72]

The symbolic codes of these stories were common knowledge. They signified the unfortunate and difficult social transitions of modernity. Such cultural challenges could only be expressed in social codes, especially in the case of suicides so that the burial tradition could be carried on. Only in the 1960s did the papers begin reporting suicides again.[73] In the early 2000s the news reporting of suicide reappeared in a different cast as journalists began to take note of the extreme suicide rates among women in Batman. When they went to collect stories for their news reports, however, they discovered silence.

Families don't talk. Even though they cannot understand the reason for their daughter's suicide, they agree that silence is the best response.[74]

That is all. She does not say a word more. However, Nurcihan's neighbors tell a different story. . . . Nurcihan burned herself with a gallon of gas exactly a month ago. The mother, Makbule, says there is nothing to tell.[75]

Just like the other girls in Batman, Diyarbakır and Muş, the cause of suicide for Gülcan, who died at the age of only seventeen, was left hidden under white paint. The wall was first washed and then painted white. [It was] as if she had never lived; all was silent, nothing was spoken.[76]

The Batman suicides were alarming. The Ministry of the Family had published a report "On Suicides and Suicide Attempts in the Official Records of the Province of Batman (1995–2000)"[77] that revealed that at least a few women had committed suicide every month from the mid-1990s onward.

Three-quarters of the suicides and suicide attempts were by women. The majority were between the ages of fourteen and thirty, and came from rural areas and low socioeconomic levels. Despite the lack of reliable data about possible causes, psychological and family-related disputes were frequently indicated. Almost 16 percent of the women were in religious marriages and 8 percent were in polygynous ones. Another study enhanced these results.[78] For example, only 72 percent of the women it surveyed were allowed to go out shopping on their own, and 84 percent were not even allowed to go to a park or a social gathering. Only 10 percent of the girls who committed suicide spoke of their depression or feelings of despair, and only 3 percent left a suicide note—86 percent departed in silence.

In addition to the patriarchal oppression that women suffered, Batman was experiencing an urbanization crisis. The region was home to ethnic unrest and clashes among the militant separatist Kurdistan Workers' Party (PKK), the Hezbollah, and the Turkish army, which had forced much of the region's rural population to abandon their homes and traditional lives and find refuge in urban centers.[79] Most lived in crowded shantytowns, and this congestion was also one of the causes of the heightened suicide rate.[80] Women typically received less than their fair share of the meager resources available.[81] While 90 percent of the families surveyed supported the education of their sons, only 20 percent supported the education of their daughters. In addition to these disheartening factors, Turkish women in general suffered from intra-family violence from parents, spouses, and siblings,[82] including violence related to "family honor." Television also played a significant role showing soap operas and other programs that depicted women with freer lives. This study concluded that the guardians of those who committed suicide in Batman had an *intuitive sense* that insult and injury experienced through relative deprivation might have been a more powerful force than the absolute deprivation that they all shared. Their suicides were an effort to "break the chains of structural/cultural/gendered oppressions."

In these lives, silence meant acceptance, and young women who lived with a desire for their own lives, even if only in their fantasy, were trapped in an *unknown*. The suicides were an exception and as an exception they revealed things about the female body in contemporary Turkey:[83] that it was oppressed, that it was silent, and that it disappeared after suicide. The exception launched significant public debate on suicide among young women. It engaged many different groups, from left-wing intellectuals to the Diyanet, from writers to feminists, in an attempt to find the social and political conditions that might have been the cause. The Nobel laureate Orhan Pamuk, for example, went to Batman after the suicide debates began, and his novel *Snow* was inspired by the life he observed there.[84] With the publication of the Batman suicide study, the story became the reference point for why women committed suicide in contemporary Turkey: anomie, inequality, sexism, terror, and violence of everyday life were among other reasons. Media attention focused on changes in women's education, yet it did not address the possibility of changing the situation by changing gender relations through educating the region's men.[85] At the same time, the media portrayed "Batman" or "the oppressive culture of the East" as the root cause of these suicides, and marginalized these female suicides in relation to suicides occurring elsewhere in the country. Observing the transplant news for many years, I was intrigued with the way suicide could be marginalized like this whereas the archetype of Ebru's suicide and subsequent organ donation had happened in the middle of Istanbul only three years prior to the debates on Batman and was celebrated as a heroic deed. Suicide had become a central biopolitical tool for the state to transform its subjects, invent alienation as in the case of Batman's bodies, or internalize the legendary female body through rites of diffusion to provide the biopolis with donors.

Diyanet's response to suicides must also have changed since the early days of the republic. Their burial was not only legitimized, but they were actually seen as victims and no longer sinners:

> There are various reasons for these suicides, such as the terrorist activities of the PKK and Hezbollah, inequalities in the distribution of income, longing for a luxurious life, culture shock, identity crises, low education level, the pressures families have over their daughters, the number of children in a household, the early marriage age for women, and superstitions that have nothing to do with religion, all of which contribute to the causes of these suicides.

> Life is a great *nimet* [blessing] from God. To kill oneself is to destroy the beauty of this *nimet*. No one has the right to do that, either by killing oneself or someone else. Only God has the right to end this *nimet*. God orders in the Qur'an (En'am 151): "Do not destroy the life God created as sacred."[86]

The response of the Diyanet to the suicides in Batman also reflected changing ideas about the place of Islam regarding matters of death and dying. People no longer lived for Islam. Instead Islam was there to help them, to provide succor and sustenance for those in need. The Diyanet constructed the Batman cases as wounds of modernization, not resistance. It spoke of these female bodies as innocent victims of modernization, and not as sinners. The religious attitude toward suicide had been very different not that long ago, especially considering issues involving burial rites. In the Hanefi tradition, suicide was considered a sin. The body belonged to God in life as in death. It would be put to sleep at burial after the departure of the *jann*, which had been given to the human from God's *nefes* (breath), and then God would restore the same breathless body to life on the Day of Judgment. Because of this, nobody was allowed to exercise power of determination over life he or she did not own. In this tradition, *life* was the *relationship* with God; and the body was the *object*, the vehicle, of this relationship.[87]

Suicide violated this sacred relationship. But from the point of view of the Diyanet, the violation seemed insignificant because these souls did not intend it; rather, they had become victims of vicious circumstances that had taken over them. The violation did not stem from within but was top-down instead. One could extend the same logic to the suicides whose organs were used for transplants, although the episodes did not entail the same bodies and were not acted out in similar regions. They, too, were victims of social life, and transplants could eventually restore their sin into a good deed by saving patients' lives. This way, the medical establishment and the media were bringing the transplant patient to health while restoring the remembrance of the suicide. With organ harvesting from suicides, technology began to replace religious hegemony over the domain of death. As a nontraditional, transformative medium, it began shaping struggles like those among Eldegez, Haberal, Kalayoğlu, and Dr. S. over the sourcing of kidneys for transplantation.

With Ebru's drama and ritual, the state could begin connecting the worlds of the media, the public, and medicine for biopolitical ends. It was not for no reason that Eldegez viewed organ transplantation as a three-part mosaic.[88] To him, only one piece was medicine; the other parts were the media and the public. He believed that of the three, the public was the most open-minded about organ donation. Utilizing the other two along with public support, he was be able to produce an image that seemed desirable for all parties involved in the making of the transplanted body and its heroic donors. While the anatomists were stuck in the liminal phase, dissecting the cadavers of the homeless and unwilling to talk about it, the transplant surgeons were able to invent a legend to "re-incorporate" the cadaveric donor into social life again. In a way, Ebru's donation was a biomedical reburial; her organs were healing transplants into the social body. She, in death, had transformed the social body materially, literally. While anatomists' "dissecting the respectable cadaver" had metaphoric qualities that reached out to the poetics of the body as also deployed in the poems of Küçük İskender, the transplant legend of Ebru operated within a different meaning-making process.

The metaphoric and quasi-literal affect of technology was symptomatic. To understand it I searched for a place that would allow me to go deeper into the semiology of space, time, and the self where I could trace how language and image worked through rites and rituals. These constituted the essence of cultural techniques, which had also been utilized for biopolitical ends. For example, Küçük İskender's poetry was evocative for anatomists. His metaphors of the cadaver, the body, and its parts seemed to transport anatomists to the outskirts of social life, confirming their vocational experience and helping them think further about anatomy, the mentally ill, and the respectable cadaver. To understand the place of internal organs in culture and the transfer of meaning in metaphors and images, I began looking into contemporary art in Turkey. That was how I met the artist Nazif Topçuoğlu, who had been using viscera as a medium in his photographs. He thought that what became alive in poetics of the body was dying in pictures that aimed to use organs as metaphors for social critique. He thought his work with organs failed to bring the messages across; for some cultural reason, where words rhymed, the image was failing.

DYING METAPHORS

Nazif Topçuoğlu hoped that when he used organs and body parts of animals to invent metaphors, it would take the message from these already highly coded objects to other places in the outskirts of social life to serve as a critique of social life. That was why he looked for metaphors embodied in flesh and blood. During an interview, he told me, "It [has been] fashionable to use blood and flesh for artistic purposes for the past ten years at least. It goes well in the [art] market. Artists freeze cadavers and exhibit [them] in freezers. They use the Visible Human Project. Marc Quinn used his own blood to sculpt his head.[89] Nothing is sacred anymore. The sacred is being pushed to its limits. Everything was so calm in Turkey. I asked myself: what can I show the public that they will respond to? Well, they did respond, but it all took time."

These were the questions occupying his mind and his art when he returned from the United States in the mid-1990s. It was then that he decided to use animal organs as media. But the organs eventually wearied him: "The metaphors emptied out—[there is] nowhere to go to with objects that signify the obvious. . . . One thinks that organs have such metaphoric power. When one speaks of the heart or the brain and other organs, it is obvious what one is referring to, right? It is so obvious that it becomes empty right away. See, for example, here I have put the brain in a box and wrapped it up with a string. My title is 'Freedom of Thought' [*Düsünceye Özgürlük*]."

He skipped through the photographs he was showing me. "In the other image I used hearts in hammocks. I call it 'Lonely Hearts.'" He moved on to another image.

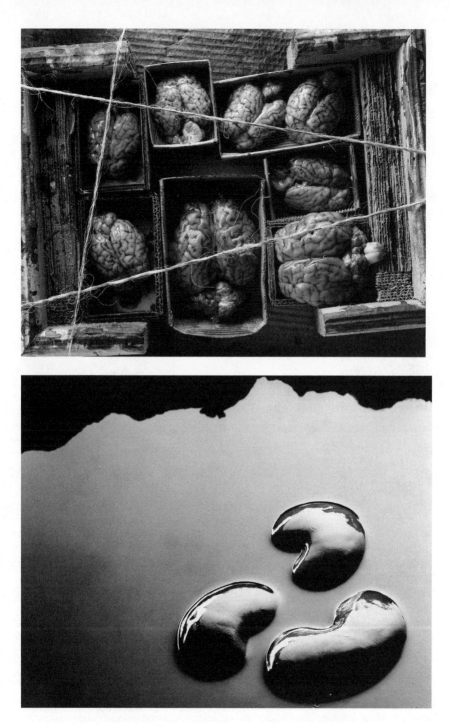

9. "Freedom of Thought." and 10. "Bean-Shaped Islands." Collection of the artist, © Nazif Topçuoğlu. Courtesy of the artist.

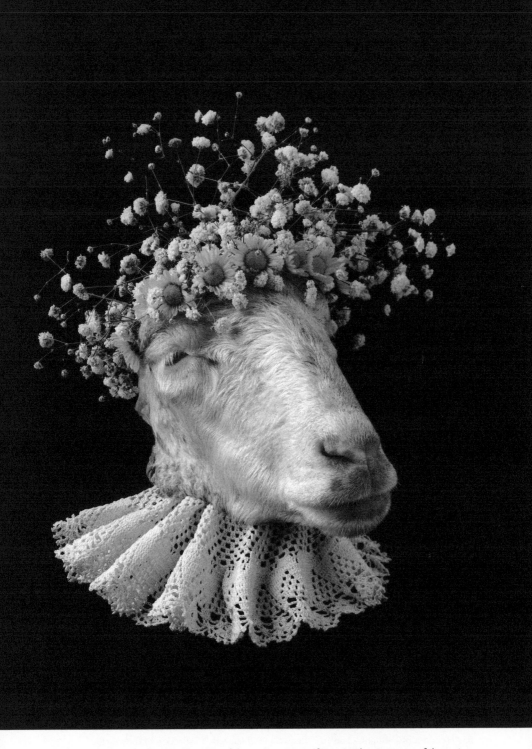

11. "Aug. 17, 1999." Collection of the artist, © Nazif Topçuoğlu. Courtesy of the artist.

These kidney images were inspired by a poem I read once, "The Bean-Shaped Island." I put them in blood, which is a thicker substance and reflects the images of the islands [the kidneys] much stronger than water would. So this is a combination of blood and kidneys and they represent the islands and the shoreline. It is the map of Istanbul. . . . The message a photograph relates to the public is in its context. An image makes no sense unless it is a document of something. It is true of the way I am interested in organs. I ask myself, what is beneath the surface? That is why I have been using viscera. In reality you cannot see beneath the organs. In the nineteenth century, when surgery began, the church was against all such operations. Roland Barthes says he has seen an analogy between photography and surgery for this reason. One cuts into the body to see it better; that is what photography should do.

Of all the photographs Topçuoğlu showed me, he was most proud of one. It was the head of a sheep adorned with bridal veil decorations, a crown of dried daisies and a lace collar. He fell in love with the head when he spotted it while browsing for body parts in a butcher shop. The head had white, wooly hair with no discoloration or dirt. It was as white and pure as a bride, he thought when he saw it. The virgin bride meant sacrifice, literally, and the photograph did not need much naming. He modeled the head to make a statement on the earthquake of 1999: "There is a saying in Turkish, 'To wait for death like a sacrificial sheep' [kurbanlık koyun gibi beklemek]. That is what I wanted to bring across; that we are waiting for the next big earthquake to come and take our lives, and we are as beautiful as newly wedded brides [who] are waiting like sheep, which wait to be sacrificed. That was my main motivation while making this bridal sheep's head." Topçuoğlu's art understood sacrifice as something that connected people to a very frail yet humane part of themselves deep down. "To wait like a sacrificial sheep" was an unspoken side of human nature. It transformed the innocent into an "offering," as a pure sacrificial victim, especially the female body in its cultural context. When this innocent offering entered the world as a sacrifice it would be consumed as flesh—a body part or an organ—and become a mediating object between the worlds of the sacred and the profane. Sacrifice was evocative. Sacrificial sheep even more so.

Traditionally the sacrifice connected worlds once a year during a ritual and reminded people of the deceased, mortality, and death. For this reason, the inside of an animal was not a taboo or unfamiliar sight to Turkish people, who from an early age routinely watched animals be ritually killed, and their organs removed and cleaned. This familiar image of organ extraction was a central part of the cultural understanding of redemption. People drew analogies between animal and human organs because of this ritualistic association. On more than one occasion, I heard analogies drawn among patients. And once an organ donor described to me in detail the insides of his body and how the surgeons must have operated on him—a knowledge he had acquired, he said, from the time he worked as a butcher. Even though, as the story tells, animals have replaced humans as sacrificial victims since the time of İbrahim, Topçuoğlu, like the ex-butcher organ donor, was at ease using them in analogy.

For Topçuoğlu, the metaphor of the offering was limited by its strong cultural overdetermination associated with the place of sacrifice in cultural life. In a way, the organs and body parts were offerings that could not exceed their specific cultural contexts. "Sacrificial brides" and other images of organs could not help him achieve the "infinite possibilities of being,"[90] which was the characteristic of art as a unifying act. On the contrary, the worlds he wanted to unite within the work of art—the self and politics— he thought, were falling apart. Internal organs and butchering were impressions of sacrifice, a ritual that unified worlds in such a sacred way that it was difficult to take meaning away from this central ritual and reinvent or rename the organs to allow metaphors to grow. In most photographs the image of the flesh had become a dead metaphor. Cutting the flesh was cutting into nothing. Juxtaposing images of flesh with other objects from the imaginary was either radically provocative or meaningless.

Why then had the image of the bridal sheep worked so well compared to the others? What kind of a cultural place did the donor occupy in a sacrificial ritual that was hard to liberate its organs from? In Topçuoğlu's artistic concerns, in transplant patient's stories of exchange, and in the semantics of the word *bağış* deployed both for transplants and sacrifice ritual, I began to understand the cultural challenges related to the invention of a suicide donor. This lifeless self could be utilized to complete the rites of passage. The elements and mechanisms of the sacrifice ritual were an essential process of redemption. Mobilized for this end, it could become the voice of the biopolis, a heroic biopolitical instrument to transform Ebru into a legendary donor.

The legend of Ebru did not transform the public image of transplants from cadaveric donors, but it helped change, even if very slightly, the number of donations and marked the suicide's donation as a historic turning point. Yet, the invention of legend took place in a culture where something very affecting about the human psyche was acting in relation with exchange and *jann*. This human condition was traditionally ritualized in the redemption process of sacrifice, a ritual we all knew so well.

SACRIFICE

Kurban—sacrifice—is the performance of a drama, a test of love between God and humans. Inspired by the story of İbrahim, it occupies a central place in Islam's religious rituals that bridged this world and beyond, the living and the dead. [91]

Sacrifice was practiced all around the Middle East in the pre-Islamic era, and later on it was incorporated into Islam as a core religious practice.[92] It could take many forms: the fulfillment of a wish, for rain or good luck, or the warding off of accidents. For example, on May 6 in Anatolia people celebrate the holiday of Hıdrelez. When nature is blooming at its peak and trees are fresh and green, it is believed that two saints, Hızır and İlyas, visit the material world to receive petitions.[93] People wander through the woods and attach to tree branches slips of paper with their prayers written on them for these saints to find. When these wishes are fulfilled, an animal is typically sacrificed to show gratitude. This folk tradition resembles other personal sacrifices that were performed to thank God for fulfilled prayers: a marriage proposal, a loved one's safe return from military service, recovery from an illness, or a healthy birth.[94] Hatice, for example, had fulfilled her sacrifice vow as soon as she had the transplant.

Wish fulfillment sacrifices were unique to individuals' experiences. They were spiritually anchored in the collective religious realm, linking individuals to social life and its echo in the void of its past. The collective celebrations of sacrifice had a grander scale. They were meant to open a dialogue with supernatural forces within the sociality of the cosmic clock;[95] they were bound to time, to the recurring memory of a story and the imaginary that the story allowed people to enter. Kurban Bayramı, the Festival of Sacrifices, was one such collective form. It is celebrated throughout the Muslim world on the tenth through the twelfth days of the month of the *Hac* (in English, Hajj), the pilgrimage to Mecca. Its most significant performance is in Mecca, home of İbrahim and Muhammad. As the story has been told in Turkey, God wanted to test İbrahim's loyalty and demanded he sacrifice his son, İsmail. Did İbrahim know God well enough, love Him enough, trust Him enough? Would İbrahim sacrifice his only son, İsmail, with whom he had been blessed at a late age, to God? While İbrahim was meditating on what to do, Satan whispered in his ear that he should doubt God and not obey him. Yet, despite Satan's intervention, İbrahim decided to obey God and kill his own flesh and blood. God, in return, showed mercy to İbrahim. He forgave İbrahim's ambivalence under Satan's influence and provided a ram to be sacrificed in İsmail's place. The literal nature of the human sacrifice was thus made symbolic, making İbrahim's story a ritual drama. As a reminder of this diabolical interference, the stoning of Satan had become a central ritual of the *Hac* (Hajj) and a central theme in people's relationship with the divine. Pilgrims on the *Hac* go to Mina, near Mecca, to ritually rebuke the devil by throwing pebbles at three walls called the *jamarat* and thereby show their faith in God. It was in Mecca where Muhammad, like İbrahim in Ur, broke the idols, and resanctified the black stone of the Kabaa, which originally had been found and installed by İbrahim and İsmail.

More than anything, İbrahim's story initiated the possibility of wish fulfillment. It framed a drama of attaining love, trust, and forgiveness by releasing what one possessed and held dear. One learned that by surrendering to the divine, one would acquire a true personal knowledge of God. İbrahim's sacrifice of his own son's body meant releasing himself into the void and consequently acquiring a new relationship with the creator. With this trusting knowledge, a faithful Muslim's place in the world was rejuvenated and socially restored. While the big collective ceremony takes place in Mecca, throughout the Muslim world every household sacrifices an animal as best can be afforded in İbrahim's memory, a microcosmic ritual mimicking İbrahim's surrender to God's command. In Turkey, butchers used to go from door to door. In the backyards of their homes, families would gather around the animal they were about to sacrifice. People observed the unwilling animals, screaming, struggling, drawing back from the tree from which they would be hung as if they knew what was about to happen.

The butcher would initiate the sacrifice with prayers. Then, after the rites were completed, the sadness in the air would be washed away and people would begin treating it like the meat they consumed everyday. The animal's organs would be taken out, washed, and prepared for special meals. Some of the meat would be kept for the family, but most of it would be sent to the poor as charity. This meat was called *bağış*, meaning "donation," the same term that is used to describe organ donation, *organ bağışı*.

The ritual concluded with a feeling of relief and contentment that what was once exclusive and personal had been shared and made collective. Sins were forgiven. *Bağış* also meant redemption, signaling the desire to be forgiven by surrendering to God. The term also underlined the ritual process through which people internalized the İbrahimic drama, subduing feelings of ownership in favor of letting go. Donation, destruction, consumption, and purification were a collective search for the forgiveness of the divine. Through these aspects, the process restored a troubled memory or assuaged a guilty conscience—a response to the appearance of a loved one in a dream or the transformation of an innocent wish into desire. With the collective dramatization of İbrahim's great sacrifice, real life experiences were brought under control. The ritual's participants were thus crucial to its conduct and completion. They gave meaning to the process. For there was always an undone, unfinished, incomplete story, a sin to be purified with the blood of the animal that flew into that individually experienced void.

Sacrifice nourishes the living. Early anthropological studies understood that the significance of sacrifice lay in the roles played during the ritual process. In traditional rituals, always a sacrifier (a priest, or in this case an imam), a sacrificer (the celebrant for whom the sacrifier works), and a sacrifice (the animal or symbol sacrificed) together opened a dialogue with the sacred.[96] Generally, the purpose of the sacrifice determined the roles of the participants, yet there were no strict definitions: the sacrificer could be the same person as the sacrifier, for example.[97] In Kurban Bayramı there was no need for an imam to initiate each single ritual because the butcher knew the prayers that allowed him to kill the animal. Yet only through the presence of those who had been authorized to pray over the killing—imam, butcher, priest—could the dialogue with the sacred be opened. These individuals could initiate and complete the ritual process; their prayers mediated between animal and human *jann*. The family, or one family member with a special prayer or petition, was the sacrifier. The sacrifier wished to restore a communication between the person, the deceased person's memory, and God. The sacrifice was complete when the butcher's knife and his prayers released the victim's blood. The animal's *jann*, or life energy, was a transforming medium connecting this world and the next in the parallel world of the ritual process. The life of the animal—its *zoë*—departed this way. Through the *jann* of the animal, the memory of the deceased was evoked and one entered the realm of the *unknowable*. The *jann* was released to restore purity. And as this happened, the animal's corpse was broken down, carved into organs and cuts of meat to be consumed later on in a festive family dinner.

According to Homeric poems, the gods consumed the meat of the animals sacrificed at their altars.[98] Sometimes the priests ate a share as well. It was believed that by consuming the victim's flesh one took a divine share, consuming what the gods consumed. The identity of the victim determined how the corpse was consumed. If the impulse to donation inspired the sacrifice, consumption made it meaningful, carrying petitions into the *unknowable*.[99]

One could hear echoes of İbrahim's great sacrifice in the stories of organ transplants from suicides, reflected back off the steel surgical instruments and legalities of biotechnological life. There were echoes in the word "donation"; in the release from bondage and ownership; in the collective consumption of the meat; in its exchange value as an emptied object communicating between the living and the divine.

In this sense, Ebru's drama followed İbrahim's story. It incorporated the character of traditional sacrifice to restore the personhood of the suicide. When Ebru's vital organs were donated to transplant patients, they were consumed like a sacrificial victim's flesh, a commodity in the making. Her internal organs restored her place in social life, which itself had become the *unknowable*—the sovereign domain no longer of God but of the biopolis. Her impure act was forgiven with the donation.

The transplant could become a possibility of redemption because of a reference in the Qur'an. A nephrologist from Cerrahpaşa University Hospital had told me of how the Diyanet cited the sura Maide (Al-Maeda, sura 5) where it gave consent to harvest organs: "Whoever keeps [a human being] alive, it is as though he kept alive all men" (5:32). The Diyanet, the physician said, supported this and glorified the donors who transplanted the donated organs of loved ones who had died through suicide.[100] By saving one soul's life one actually saved the whole world. By saving the life of a patient, one could be redeemed of all sin, even from the greatest sin of all, suicide. "This," the nephrologists told me the Diyanet claimed, "will give these poor people a chance to go to God's heaven in spite of the fact that they committed suicide. Saving a life is like saving the world."[101]

To Be Sacrificed

In 2002, Merve, a woman in her early twenties, committed suicide in Istanbul. She jumped from the tenth floor of her apartment building one morning while her husband was at work. The note she left was not only a testimony of her pain, but a will addressed to her family and to the transplant doctors.

> [To her husband:] I wish I could tell you not to feel guilty for my suicide, but you should. . . . I cannot endure this life any longer. So I have to die. I am afraid I will go mad. Take care of our daughter. . . . She is a part of you. . . . I asked you that we should move out of this apartment. This apartment is calling me to death. Do you know how it feels to pray for death every day? I lived only for our baby until now. But my body is destroyed. But now my soul shall be with me.

> [To her mother:] Mom, I begged you to rescue me, I told you I was feeling so bad. I told you either I will go crazy here or kill myself. You left me alone. . . . But please do not leave my daughter alone. Please do not have them send her to the village. . . . And do not make any ritual *duas* [prayers] and *mevlüt* [birth and burial rites] for me. Do not. . . . Do for once just as I wish. And do not donate my organs, because I love them. Let them rot with me.[102]

Did Merve know the legend of Ebru? No one can say. She must have known that the organs of suicides were being used for transplants. She must have thought about how she could remain herself in death without being appropriated for the social body. Her suicide made the headlines of a small newspaper, *Posta*, but it was not mentioned in any of the large national papers. With the legend of Ebru, a sin was redeemed and turned into something positive and normal, transforming suicide into sacrifice. Merve, in contrast, was trying to create for herself a space and an identity where she could be complete in the integrity of her own body, a whole person. She had no regrets for what she was about to do. A transplant surgeon told me in response to Merve's story, "We are becoming tired of living in this society. And that is what Merve is telling us, no? She says 'I am not giving you my life, I do not agree with your customs, I do not believe in your system, I do not agree with the way you live or make me live.' She is a marginal. There are people like her. She hates her life; why would she want to give her organs?"

To donate organs, then, one had to love life, community, society, traditions; one had to share the body with what one shared love. Merve, in contrast, attempted to retain her self by shrinking into her body; she tried to remain a *homo sacer*, a person who could not be touched or included in the normal order of life because she was impure.[103] *Homo sacer*—Latin for "sacred man"—could not be judged, punished, or cleansed because of having interfered with and acted against the divine order; no human should indeed be allowed to interact with this contaminating figure. Merve's testimony was an effort to preserve this condition, her sovereignty. It even reached beyond that to make a political statement: prayers and organ donation should not be held for her, the *homo sacer* who longed for exclusion from social life in order to keep her self intact.

With the invention of the suicide donor as a life-less object in the biopolis, *homo sacer* became a *homo sacrem* in the hands of transplant surgeons. Ebru's organs were desirable charitable offerings. As gifts, they reincorporated her into the pure and clean order of Muslim life while making her a legend for saving other people's lives. Her blood shed by her own hand became the basis for her spiritual salvation, but in truth it was merely appropriated to provide biological salvation to the recipients of her organs and prestige and status to transplant surgeons being weighed on the scales of modernity. The elements hidden in the metaphor of suicide as sacrifice were sufficient to naturalize transplant technology. Merve's story taught me where the pulse of social life beat. It was in the resistance against loss of communication, love, and care all secretly enveloped in the metaphors of a most traditional and central ritual, the sacrifice. There people came to terms with each other by giving up on their most cherished thing to the divine, their lives.

Self-Sacrifice

İntihars means self-sacrifice in Arabic, a meaning lost in its translation into Turkish. The history of the word in Turkish shows that it dates back to the Tanzimat in the early days of Ottoman modernity. Traditionally *kendini katletmek*, "to kill oneself," was used instead. According to Arkun, İntihar has Arabic roots—the Arabic *"nahr,"* or sacrifice.[104] Throughout the ages, the drama of self-sacrifice has changed form, taking lives, revealing oppressive experiences, displaying possibilities of life and death.

The Turkish playwright Güngör Dilmen Kalyoncu's *Kurban* (sacrifice, 1979) appropriated the theme of Euripides' play *Medea*, which was translated into Turkish in the 1950s by Ahmed Hamdi Tanpınar. *Kurban* was inspired by *Medea* but adapted to Turkish culture, referencing both ancient Greek and modern Turkish theater and unifying İbrahim's great sacrifice and self-sacrifice.[105] *Kurban* dramatized the life of a peasant woman in rural Anatolia, re-narrating *Medea*'s terrifying replacement of a sacrificial ritual with the sacrifice of the peasant woman's own children and her own suicide.

Güngör Dilmen Kalyoncu's *Kurban* is the story of a married couple, Mahmud and Zehra, who live in the village of Karacaören in Anatolia, in present-day Turkey. The couple has been married for over ten years, but now Mahmud wants to take a second wife. What is more, he wants to marry her in an official, state-sanctioned ceremony instead of just a religious ceremony like the one in which he and Zehra were married. In the first act, their two young children, Murat, nine, and Zeyneb, four, play with a ram that is to be sacrificed the next day when their father brings home Gülsüm, his new wife. The children complain to their father that they love the ram and do not want to see the new bride. Mahmud tries to comfort his children by telling them that it is an important tradition he has to follow, that it will all be fine when Gülsüm is there, and that it is a good thing that God will accept the life of the ram. "In the ancient times," he tells his children, "men had to sacrifice their loved ones to God." The children want to hear the story so he goes on.

> Once there lived this prophet, İbrahim. He had only one child, İsmail, whom he adored more than anything else in the world, like I adore you. One day God spoke to him: "İbrahim, I have given you the son

you wished for in your late age, and now I want him back. I want you to sacrifice him to me." So İbrahim takes İsmail to the mountains to sacrifice him there. On the way up to the mountain, he prays silently to know what he should do. As the road ends and İbrahim is alone with İsmail, he asks İsmail if he is afraid. İsmail says no. So he blindfolds his son and takes his knife out. Still he is debating with himself—what if it was not God but Satan who was speaking to him? Then he would be committing a great sin and would be killing his one and only son. However, he decides to follow his heart. Just as he is about to kill him, God speaks again. "No, İbrahim, enough, you have proven to me your loyalty. I do not want İsmail's blood. You and İsmail are free." And so God brought down a beautiful ram from the sky to be sacrificed instead of İsmail.[106]

Mahmud ends his story, telling his children that God has sent the ram as a gift to replace the children in the sacrifice, and so the children should not pity it.

That night Gülsüm's brother Mirza visits the family to make the final arrangements for the wedding. He starts arguing with Mahmud over the *başlık parası*, the dowry. Mirza wants Mahmud and Zehra's most fruitful piece of land in exchange for his sister. Mahmud is not willing to give it up. The argument goes on for a little while. Zehra sits in the other room, listening in sadness. She remembers the first time she met Mahmud—how much they loved each other, how they married and worked hard to buy that land. Everything is falling apart in her little world with the coming of the new bride; she listens to Mahmud speak of Gülsüm and her beauty, bargaining with their own land. Mirza is not willing to accept anything but the land for the bride price, and Mahmud gets angry and kicks him out. The deal is broken.

While Mahmud is talking to Mirza, Zehra meets some neighbors in front of her house. She tells them how sad she is that Mahmud is taking a new wife from the neighboring village. They have all heard the news already. They have all been there. They share her sadness and promise to tell Mahmud he should think it over and not let his happy marriage be damaged. Mahmud walks Mirza out, and on his way back home he meets an elderly woman who tells him not to marry Gülsüm, not to cause such pain to his wife. Mahmud gets angry. But when he gets back home, his mind seems to be already made up. Despite Gülsüm's beauty, he does not want to give away all that he has. The price is too high.

At home, Mahmud finds Zehra dressed in her wedding gown. Her hair is down, and she speaks in gentle, chanting words. Mahmud apologizes to Zehra and says he did not mean to hurt her. He says he thought Gülsüm could be a good co-mother to their children and help Zehra around the house. But as they speak and Zehra tells Mahmud how much she loves him, he keeps thinking of Gülsüm. His passion for her is beyond his love for his wife. He cannot remain faithful to Zehra, despite their history together. At that moment Mahmud makes up his mind: "You should prepare the ram for sacrifice in the morning," he tells Zehra. "I will bring Gülsüm home."

That night Zehra dreams of her neighbors, the women of the village. They appear in her room carrying Gülsüm's corpse. At first she does not understand what is happening. The women tell her that they killed her to make Zehra happy. They put the corpse next to Mahmud while he is asleep to scare him and to make him appear guilty of the murder. Zehra is shocked. She wants the corpse out of their home, but just at that moment the *muhtar*, the village headman, appears. He has heard gunshots and wants to know what is going on. Zehra looks at Mahmud and Gülsüm in the bed together and sees the young woman moving. She is not dead. Gülsüm has awakened, the women say; she came back to life by Mahmud's love. Mirza walks in with the *muhtar* to find his sister in Mahmud's bed. It is against the traditions, but if the power of love is so strong then it is all right to kidnap a woman, he says. Zehra is left all alone.

She wakes up the next morning and tells her children to take the ram to the meadow and release it. The children are very happy. They think they will not have a stepmother and the ram's life will be saved. They return to the house filled with joy. Zehra makes them some tea, mixing it with opium to make them fall asleep. Then she locks the gate of the house. Shortly after, Mahmud arrives and knocks on the door. There is no answer. He calls for Zehra but there seems to be no one at home. Gülsüm is with him, along with all of her village, ready to start the wedding celebrations. But they need to sacrifice the ram first. So they look for the ram in the stable and around the house, but it is nowhere to be found. One of the neighbors tells them that the children have set it free. Just then, Zehra appears on the balcony of the house. She tells Mahmud that she will not accept the new bride, nor will Gülsüm become a stepmother to their children. Mirza wants to get into the house by force, but Zehra tells him she will kill their children if any of them come in. Mahmud and Mirza begin to argue. Mahmud tries in vain to calm Zehra down. As Mirza and the other villagers decide to break into the house, it is already too late. Mahmud walks into his house to find his two children and his wife lying dead on the floor.

Kurban is a statement on the tragedy of polygyny and love. *Kurban*'s cultural specificity added a new layer to the drama of *Medea*. It integrated the ritualistic characteristic of sacrifice to make the drama of Zehra's resistance against polygyny more meaningful. With her husband's second marriage Zehra would lose all that binds her to this world: the land they owned together and their bond as husband and wife, which would be regarded as the unofficial marriage. Her union with her husband had come to a dead end. Her land had been exchanged for a woman who was to replace her entirely. She took her own life and the lives of her children. The significance of *Kurban* was the way this drama played out when a literal sacrifice was made. As in *Medea*, it was unclear until the final scene whether the drama was about the sacrifice indicated by the Turkish play's title. Only with the presence of the ram in the story could suicide become sacrifice. Zehra's and her children's lives were replaced with the life of the ram God sent to Earth to be sacrificed in the traditional festivities. Then the ram was set free and the children were made its substitutes. The legend of Ebru was a reversal of the story of İbrahim and İsmail, a story not of stopping human sacrifice but of reintroducing it in a high-tech setting, this time not for God, but for the sake of people. Mahmud's children were sacrificed in exchange for violating his sacred marriage bonds with his first wife, marrying against her will, and erasing her material and social sense of well-being. Zehra, like the suicides in Batman, functions as an index of unbearable social structural pressures on women cast in a religious paradigm of explanatory protest. Ebru's "liberation" took this paradigm a step further, merging it with a new ritual of diffusion of the sacred breath of life, of parts of the *emanet* body given to each human being, now redistributed to save six other lives. Ebru's sins were purified, her personhood was restored, her body parts were "in life" and she was someone who could be properly mourned and celebrated.

Both *Medea* and *Kurban* dramatized women's lives as archetypes, showing their transformations into the same structural form of "letting go of life" also encapsulated by the legend of Ebru. They shed some light on the powerful ways cultural mechanisms continue unfolding in codes slightly different in the spirit of each age. In transplants, the deployment of a suicide's body again invoked sacrifice's central theme of "redemption," this time in technoscientific settings, in rituals for transplant patients with human organs as offerings, in a virtual space of performance in the media, and in a material body given away—all these within the biopolis.

THE POSSIBLE

With the legend of Ebru, transplant surgeons had achieved a historic turning point in the number of donation cards signed for cadaveric transplants. They were able to relate to the public for the first time with respect to donations for biomedicine. Neither efforts to name brain death by different Latin or Turkish terms nor the general consent of the Diyanet had helped until then to increase the donations as significantly. Ebru's donation was a rite of passage in the biopolis; it was a rite of diffusion as she diffused into the social life, disappeared, and became invisible yet still lived through the donation of her organs. Hers was a technoscientific rite of passage, as she diffused with much public "pleasure" or *jouissance* into social life to materialize the brain-dead donor, which could not be invented simply by way of Latin or Turkish words, religion's consent, and other efforts to begin its commodification. The rite eased the invention of the technological objects and the incorporation of the human body in donor and recipient relations within the biopolis—its eased passage from one reality to another.

The two places in medicine where such rites were actually necessary to maintain an ongoing practice were cadaveric transplants and anatomy dissections. The rite of diffusion's three stages—invention, purification, and diffusion—paralleled the stages of separation, transition, and incorporation that Arnold van Gennep famously noted in rites of passage.[107] They allowed the collective to participate in a transitional phase, which could be maintained as a proper reburial for the deceased.

To begin, cadaveric transplantation and anatomy needed surplus bodies, a stable pool of donors, dead bodies. The invention of a liminal communitas was a kind of separation, a marking of social difference. This was the role of the *kadavra* or the suicide donor. Cultural stigmatization of such marginal bodies marked their difference, yet their proximity to medical practice enabled their incorporation—they were *known* to exist, they were locatable in the hospital, they bore at least the traces of social attachment, and they were vulnerable, their personhood could be restored. They could still be seen and invented as persons, and this possibility—and only this—allowed them to become a part of the rite of diffusion.

Yet without purification by traditional rituals as in sacrifice or burial ceremonies and without an accompanying discourse of compassion and regret, the diffusion of these surplus bodies would not be possible. Now desirable biomedical objects, these needed more than the biological criteria required for brain-death diagnosis or formaline to preserve their flesh. In a transitional phase, they needed society's approval and a cultural conformation so that they could materialize as technological or life-less objects to be used for medical ends. The purification discourse gave a new context and meaning to feared but much needed cadaveric donors, allowing suicides to be made a part of social life again. This way, the *jann* in these bodies was diffused into others' bodies with the transplanted organs, pure and acceptable. The same was true for anatomy. Though not as complicated a ritual as the invention of the suicide donor, the naming of "the respectable human" was a similar act of purification that would alter the corpse at least as much as formalin and make it a person again.

Once invented from local surplus bodies and purified through rituals, these bodies became medical objects somewhat diffused into the social body such that their biographies disappeared. They were incorporated back into social life in good memories despite their dramatic life histories. With their new identities, their *jann* diffused into the population. They could be transformed into life-less biomedical objects, since either their social or biological lives were regarded as incomplete.

As suicide donors could become donors for transplants, and the rite of diffusion was completed, the anatomists were trapped within the transitional phase, which could not somehow transform the mentally ill into respectable humans. The anatomists' rite of diffusion, though much needed, was incomplete. Unlike the trauma, secrecy, and invisibility inflicted and endured in anatomical dissection, surgical transplantation had a voice. It could speak to the public. It could seek salvation and thereby both purify and commodify the body. In surgeons' hands, the dead were diffused into the living giving *life*. In anatomical dissections, the aborted rite of passage was traumatic because the rite of diffusion was inverted, asocial, not public. Anatomists created "respectable" cadavers from the unclaimed bodies of the mentally ill, but they practiced in a hospital basement, next to the memory of a pool of the dead, and far from sight. Transplant surgery operated at a different level; though it too commodified the dead body, it cured and gave life to the ill. With the help of the sacrificial restoration of organ harvesting, it successfully reincorporated the dead into its practice as "heroes" and "heroines." By making the "impure" into a biomedical object, transplant surgery completed the rite of diffusion for the living. With diffusion, the suicide was restored to acceptable memory, and its *jann* lived on in the social body. This diffusion paralleled the commodification process inherent in objects of trade.

All similar objects had to be restored into "humane" objects to be acceptable as objects of trade and medicine. By "humane" I do not mean the glorification of the donors and their tragic biographies, but on the contrary the new identities inscribed to them so that physicians continued their dialogue with patients in a kind of normalcy. When patients internalized these objects they did not internalize excluded biographies, but rather things that would become functional and unremarkable parts of their selfhood in their inner world, inside them. Transforming the cadaver into a "respectable human" would ease medical students into a respectable education, medicine itself. Transforming the suicide into a brain-dead donor would evoke sacrifices made to keep human life going. Transforming allografts into objects of trade with no trace of life or biography left in them, appearing on the hospital shelves as if fallen from the sky, would provide matrixes in abundance for the immediate and increasing demand for orthopedic surgery without confrontation with the world of the dead sleeping in the warm earth at home or in foreign lands.

These life-less objects were made into things with which one could engage as if they were objects of exchange from living bodies. The rites of diffusion allowed their passages to our lives as living memories. An object was always half coming right out of the lab. Clinical trials, human experiments, the ethical guidelines of the U.S. National Institutes of Health, and the U.S. Food and Drug Administration or other similar approvals were ontological, ethical, and epistemic elements that allowed their production as commodities in international networks of trade. Yet, to become internal objects, they first had to be absorbed into social life through names, rites, rituals, legends, and myths. Then, they could acquire some life, some identity, some thing that one could relate to. Patients internalized this part of objects too: the second half of their meaning. I, too, have tried here to interpret this *Other* half of life-less objects constructed upon political and medical histories to understand how they function in the modern Turkish biopolis, a virtual, psychic, and cultural space.

Like a shiny coin half leaning yet propped up on Earth, held up through invisible relations among elements of our ever changing, tangible, material world. This was how I began to view the biopolis and the affects of bio-medical technologies.

CONCLUSION

NEW LIFE

As I began meeting transplant patients, I was intrigued by their unusual psychic transitions. Patients were talking of a universe that had made profound impressions on them: they were reasoning with life, thinking about ethics, considering buying a kidney, rethinking their intimate relationships at home, utilizing life from all corners of society to maintain normalcy but also to give meaning to their conditions. They were changing in response to the invisible threats that constituted the new biopolis into which they were entering. My ethnography has tried to single out these relationships, to see each of them separately, so that I can follow them to the objects to which they led and to the people they affected, and to see how they were linked to one another in such a logic that one believed it to have, in Lévi-Strauss's words, an "explosion of truth," thus experiencing their dilated meanings.

EPISTEMIC PASSAGES

I have gone from site to site for this reason, to be able to share the impressions of my fieldwork: the hospital room with many dialysis machines; paired operating rooms with a patient in one room prepared to receive a kidney from the donor in the next room; a private office for a physician also known as the organ mafia; an intensive care unit (ICU) with many people lying detached from the world around them, attached to machines, staring into the void and breathing; a meeting room with a desk laden with catalogues for human bones (in English); another meeting room with many pictures of Atatürk on the wall and a burly transplant surgeon sitting underneath; a cold and damp dissection room with four tables, four cadavers, three mirrors, a standing skeleton, and a sink basin; a courtyard in a mental hospital where people meet to drink tea, smoke, and play backgammon; a buried Byzantine cemetery underneath the mental hospital; a Muslim cemetery with old and new gravestones extending into the aesthetics of life through leaves and grass, nearby a mosque, a shrine, a place for sacrifices, and open-air book stalls filled with sacred and popular religious texts.

In retrospect my fieldwork was like an "epistemic passage" moving me from one stage of knowing the world to another through a set of transferences. In each step, I attempt to understand the object relations from their invention to their internalization. These passages revealed life and people, anthropology and my place in it. When in 2000, I joined a team of anthropologists with Organs Watch, led by Nancy Scheper-Hughes and Lawrence Cohen at the University of California, Berkeley, I began to study organ trafficking in Turkey as part of a big project to map the routes of the global illegal organ trade, a technical effort to map a topography of institutions often thought of as the "underground." But during that fieldwork, I met Dr. S. and became acquainted with the world that he inhabited, and my own intellectual and emotional world slowly began to change. It was not, as one might guess, this man's vanity, his arrogance, his ambitious and wild imagination, or the cruelty of his justifications that could have caused this to happen. It was rather the wider world I was allowed to visit through him, a world that was concealed behind the terms we use in our everyday discourse, terms like capitalism, globalism, and the world order. There, I realized that the "underground" was not really under ground, and public health institutions were not merely health-care providers. In a global world capital flew in many directions with much complexity and fragmentation; localities mattered as much as individual characters. I began to see this complex emerging technological world as a universe in its own right, and that is why I called it the biopolis in this book. Patients were mobilized to find a "kidney" within it; there they also learned how to speak of their bodies, their illnesses, the kidneys, the dialysis machine, their daytime visions and their nightmares, all filled with the physical and psychic liveliness of the biopolis that had to emerge from within their own traditions and language.

Back then, I spent most of my time in Istanbul, a city to which I would return several times over the years in the course of writing this book. Istanbul was home to many transplant units but also home to a long and sometimes tiresome history. As the dark blue waters of the straits run from the Russian Black Sea to the warmer climes of the Mediterranean, big ships carrying ideologies, philosophies, and poetics, among many other goods, arrived in Istanbul, evoking the histories of the Russian Empire and the Ottoman Empire, followed by those of the Soviet Union and the Turkish Communists, of the capitalist West, and the nationalism of the modernizing Turkish secular republic. The legacy of Nazım Hikmet the poet, who died in exile in Moscow, may still be sailing in one of those ships to check on those left behind. The only "brain" Dr. Osman had owned for dissection had arrived on a ship such as this from Moscow. Bünyamin, the main character in İhsan Oktay Anar's novel *Puslu Kıtalar Atlası*, discussed in part 1, would look for secret anatomical drawings in ships sailing from Italy four hundred years ago. People, too, arrived. Laborers, prostitutes, or businessman who were all in the "business of life." Patients could view the density of traffic of these ships from Pierre Loti Hill at the top of Eyüb Sultan, where they might be having a cup of tea and viewing the Golden Horn through the centuries-old leaning gravestones. Maybe they would initiate a small sacrifice down in the foothills of Eyüb later on, or say a little prayer in the mosque while meditating on life in the deep green light reflected through the old stained glass windows.

If the sky was clear of the gray smoke of coal fires, people would appear bathed in pink and blue light reflected upon the city's old and gray buildings that have aged along with the extraordinary stories of its dense and diverse population. Life was for people, and patients, too, hold on to life to survive as they wait and hope that someday, from faraway lands or from within Istanbul's cheap modern concrete buildings, a kidney could become available. And then, they, too, would have an operation like the "lucky wealthy" people who did not have to get listed on organ allocation lists, who could pay for a donor and have Dr. S. operate on them.

Within tales of the intersecting lives of Istanbul's inhabitants, patients' destinies sometimes overlapped with human traffickers. In the dense city, the stories on crime—burglary, theft, street fights, or terrorism—were vividly told in local places where people have made Istanbul's destiny their own: at the barber shop, at the coffee house, during tea parties, in the taxicab, and in other less formal social settings. Patients talked about crime and survival strategies, naturally including organ traffickers and prominent transplant surgeons. After renal failure, some like Fidan refused to socialize because they cannot bear the thought of being entangled within such complicit circles. Oğuz thought the opposite. He wanted to become a character from the movies so that he was no longer half a human, but literally a bionic man, a "robot" as he had worded it. This way, he could fight again in the streets as he used to do with his gang—in the same neighborhood where Dr. S. used to have his office next to a small private hospital and many medical supply stores.

This part of the city, the shoreline of the Anatolian side of Istanbul, was on the exact opposite side from the Golden Horn and from Eyüb Sultan. Nazif Topçuoğlu's photo "Bean-Shaped Islands" was the map of this shoreline, kidneys representing the small Princess Islands and the blood representing the sea. On land, Dr. S. had been caught transplanting organs into Israeli recipients. In a hospital not that far away, most of the patients I had met were being treated. The culture of the flesh, traded, painted, and photographed, was a naturalized part of everyday life. What was somehow unnatural was that the patients had to internalize it, make it personal and their own. It was there in the hospital, it seemed to me, that affect emerged. Many wanted to have a transplant, soon and safely. This was why the trafficking of bodies had begun to contribute a large number of transplants, this was why patients found out about travel agencies, foreign countries, and other options. Physicians encouraged patients to search for a cure abroad if there was no match in the family. Only some had been lucky enough to be able to have a transplant from a family member, but even that was an easier success medically than psychologically.

A kidney from a family member or an unrelated loved one could transform that relationship into a tyrannical one. Oğuz had chronic rejection and a personality change after receiving his father's kidney. Zehra could not believe that the man who gave her his kidney was her real biological father. Hatice had her sister's kidney, which she felt obliged to keep as healthy as if she were taking care of her sister for the rest of her life. Sedat had become a tyrant at home after the English physician imposed Sedat's wife's kidney on him. He had organ rejection three years later. Fidan's siblings had offered her money so that she could buy herself a kidney, but that was not actually what she had hoped for. What was an "easy form of exchange" and a surgical operation had deep and traumatic consequences that began with the questioning of the most intimate relationships.

But in the biopolis, living-related transplants were encouraged by physicians due to the low numbers of cadaveric donors. This was also backed up with scientific rationales that living related transplants had higher survival rates because there was less trauma than with an organ that was kept "alive" for a number of hours while traveling great distances. That was why dialysis patients were encouraged to speak to their family members about the possibility of a biological match within the family. This required delicacy, a fine balance of intra-family relations. Then, at the same time, most of the patients would put their names on the organ-sharing waiting list. If their financial circumstances were strong enough, like Aziz or Sedat, they would look into health-care services abroad: they would be in the market for a kidney. All of these were immense efforts for people with ailing bodies on dialysis and nearing death. In a gradual and subtle way patients would become part of an "underground" as they began exploring the market for a kidney and with it they would internalize ethical disputes that extended to their political choices and their love for their state.

They were in the market for a kidney, if they could afford it. And true, Turkey was a hub. One emerging trade route connected Turkey with Russia, Europe, and Israel. Another was in the southeast of Turkey partly for those who had chosen to travel to India for a transplant in the early 1990s. While Nancy Scheper-Hughes found out about large routes of organ traffickers in Latin America, the United States, South Africa, the Philippines, Moldova, Turkey, and Israel, to which the wealthy could travel to purchase organs, Lawrence Cohen met organ donors in India whose suffering revealed not merely a material poverty but an impoverishment under the social pressures after the transplant. One Turkish patient loved this exotic new universe in India that gave her life, not knowing the whereabouts of the donor. Dr. S. used to provide donors from India in the 1990s, but that market became less prominent when the Indian government banned sales of organs. Demand moved to other regions, especially to Iraq, Palestine, Israel, and to the south of Turkey. By the mid-1990s, Turkish patients had begun going to Baghdad for transplants, a business that had been initiated by an organ recipient who had a transplant in Bagdat. In time this situation changed: Turkish kidney patients began going to Iraq to buy organs from Iraqis. These places, so alien and unknown, would begin to occupy patients' thoughts day and night: a transplant in India, or in Moscow, or at home, or maybe a living related kidney, or, if they were very lucky, one from a *kadavra*. With these in mind, they would evaluate their possibilities and the trade-offs of benefits and costs on the ethical plateaus of survival.

The region, before the war, was no less troubled in regard to trading labor. Its landscape hid much behind its barren mountains, as necessities like guns and drugs were procured and exchanged as parts of life and trade, linking families and tribes over the national borders and psychological boundaries. People of the region, Muslim, Christian, and Jewish, Iraqi, Kurdish, Turkish, Süryani, and Syrian, all traded but also suffered alike. In the normal flow of life through kin, traditions, and war, the transplant body was a new technological good, a new introduction. Over the past decades, political instability has disrupted visibility, concealed human disappearances, and opened new dimensions for the re-valuation of the body's insides as a profitable entity. Like the slowly disappearing borders and emerging violence in the region, the body's protective boundaries also seemed to vanish. The transparency of the living body as a medical commodity emerged under these circumstances, manifesting itself in the patients' bodies and the poor's hopes on the opposite sides of a medical deal.

In reaction to speculations of organ theft related to the organ trade, one transplant physician described to me the "natural" landscape of the biopolis in southeastern Turkey. Since the war in Iraq, there was more poverty in the Middle East than ever before and bodies were in abundance. Why then kill people for organs if you could find them in living bodies for sale? Patients desired healthy lives with new kidneys, lives with bodies that were whole and free of the bondage of dialysis. This desire sometimes mingled with international crime organizations as patients searched for kidneys, sometimes it was satisfied within a family by a donation, and sometimes it was fulfilled in a public hospital involving a private monetary deal between the patient and the donor without the surgeons' knowledge of it. The variety of forms of exchange depended on many things, from the health-care provider to the limits of morality the patient was ready to reach.

When they went on dialysis, most of the patients were encouraged to think of the "option" of buying an organ. They had heard of Robin Hood (Dr. S.), like they had heard of Israeli patients landing in Turkey for operations, or the travel agents who took people to Moscow. They meditated on this for a long time. These ethical plateaus were home to most of the technological objects patients would be introduced to in the biopolis, and the conversations with other patients as well as doctors affected patients' ideas and choices on organ sales. While on dialysis, they talked about this universe all the time. Aziz and Sedat had heard of organ sales and were mobilized. Hatice could not make up her mind about the possibility of buying an organ, while Fidan could not even think of it because of her financial circumstances. Aziz would not think of buying a kidney from a living donor on moral grounds; he would not want to take advantage of a poor man's life. Like Aziz, Sedat had received a cadaveric organ in Moscow. Hatice bloomed when she spoke about how she had been informed about the cadaveric donor she had been given from the organ allocation program. By God's will, these cadaveric organs would grow again with the resurrecting body on the Day of Judgment. Instead of rotting in the earth they would heal transplant patients. There was a comfort related to this condition, which was in line with the proper order of how the body was related to God through life; it was as if patients' bodies continued the same relationship with God yet with another *emanet*, a kidney, from the domain of God in the cemetery. Unlike Oğuz and Zehra, who experienced deep psychoses regarding the changes in the nature of their own bodies or others' bodies, those few patients who received organs from brain-dead donors were feeling the change in a different way. They had been relieved from dialysis and could begin a new life without bondage. Oğuz and Zehra, in contrast, felt trapped in old relationships, which already had been tyrannical and obligating.

God

When patients and physicians spoke of death, it was not faith but God that they often referred to. I thought it must have been because the body's changing relationship with its creator—our profound relationship with God—occupied transplant patients' thoughts. But beyond patients' own natural deliberations on life, death, and God, physicians seemed to be occupied with similar thoughts on God. I had spent most of my time in gloomy hospital rooms, some days talking to patients and entering their private worlds as a stranger welcomed, and some days listening to physicians who felt they had to find ways to connect me to their inner lives through the sacredness of their practice. One such instance revealed a glimpse of casuistry, a deliberation on matters of life and death related to vocation. It was a symbolic performance:

While I was talking to some doctors in the common room—out of nowhere and to my surprise, for this was a very unusual monologue to begin with—Ali, a surgeon, began telling a story from the Qur'an (2:30–34): "Allah says, 'I want to create a *Halife* [literally a caliph or legate—someone to carry on his work] on Earth!' The angels reply, 'Do you want to create something that will cause *fesat* [evil, sedition] and shed blood on Earth?' Allah says, 'Don't you know my power [and wisdom]?' The angels agree—they do. Allah says, 'You can ask Adam about every named thing. He knows the names of all things; you don't have that knowledge or capacity to name.' "

Ali concluded, "The human [*insan*] represents [*temsilci*] God on Earth. And it is a monstrous creature. The strange thing, however, is that it comes from this tiny, primitive thing called the sperm. So why did God create?

His colleague responded, "Maybe from us, from our children, he can create someone who will change the world."

Ali replied with another quotation: " 'There is nothing wrong in my plan,' says God. That is why I am asking myself, why did he create me? Why did he make me a doctor?"

I was watching silently. The room was gloomy. Outside, many patients awaited the doctors' attention. The dingy setting for Ali's meditation clashed with the aura of divinity and medical idealism of his story. These physicians were romanticizing the perfectibility of nature and the power of humankind, their own power and their own place in this order. But their reality did not correspond to the loftiness of their hearts. The room, these doctors' minds, and my mind as I sat with them all seemed befogged by Istanbul's difficulties, the poverty of its people, the suffering of the patients next door, and the physicians' own despair.

Others spoke of God and creation in relation to their role in the world. One believed surgeons were like gods. "No one else in the world but surgeons has the right to cut the body into pieces and parts," he said. He had read this in the yellowed pages of a medical textbook as a freshman and he never forgot it. "God has chosen us as surgeons. He has given us permission to cut into the body. . . . Surgeons have to learn the skills and have an education, but moreover they are special people chosen to work on the body. Surgery is the most absurd profession in the world when you think about it—for this reason it could not be done without God's consent." A nephrologist made a similar comment: medicine was a holy vocation, and doctors did not need to justify their practices because they were doing divine work. One prominent transplant surgeon believed that the work of a surgeon came second only to God's: "This is how it is in Turkey, this is how it is in the world," he said smiling, bonding his vocation with an elite group of physicians operating all around the globe. Titiz, the head of Haydarpaşa Numune Hospital's transplant unit, said he felt like Prometheus after his first successful transplant operation. Likewise when Karpuzoğlu recounted for me the first time he harvested organs from a brain-dead donor and sent them off to another city for transplantation, a bright smile lit his face. "I made organs fly," he said. "The organs flew. . . . It was a miracle."

The fantastic had become reality. And so, in my mind, from then on transplant physicians shared the same powerful universe with the ancient mythic beings that occupied the dense air that had filled the old landscapes of Anatolia for centuries. From what physicians were saying, they could rule over life like these half-human and half-god beings and govern between the worlds of humans and the gods. Surgeons were transforming the *impossible*, making it a tangible reality within the limits of "reason." The people who were able to reach the closest to the God within, the closest to the *unknowable* realm God inhabited, were surgeons, opening up the body, cutting into its depths, physically operating upon a realm with their eyes and hands, and doing this every day. They could touch and manipulate it like no one else. The surgeon had claimed a rightful place almost next to God; the kidney was a loss to be filled; and life had become technology. Transplant surgery ruled with such power to transform the body's fundamental relationship with God: life itself.

Machine

It was the machine, the system, and the artificial to which transplant patients had to relate, assisted by physicians who thought of themselves as closest to God. Patients would wake up from comas to see their arms attached to dialysis machines with their blood flowing in and out. It was the first little shock, as several had called it. And after they had been told of the renal failure and that the machine was a substitute for that loss of bodily function, they had to accept this new life on the machine and get on with it. It was probably the most dramatic moment for many. Waking up from a coma, Zehra remembered that she could hardly move as she opened her eyes in the unfamiliar setting of a crowded ICU. She could not accept this "new life" for many months. The same had been the case for Hatice, who went into early labor and then woke up to see the machine next to her bedside instead of her baby. Where had they taken her? Was she well and safe? Aziz had fallen into a coma in an emergency room without knowing the root cause of his illness, imagining it was a diabetic seizure, a hereditary illness in his family. Like these patients, many others were taken to the ER when they were half-conscious. There they would open their eyes to a new life with a machine in charge of their bodies. As the machine entered patient's lives abruptly, metaphors associated with its place in culture came along with it, imposing a new sphere of life upon their privacy.

Besides the sudden trauma of a new beginning on the dialysis machine, patients must have had a difficult time trying to make sense of something they hardly had a relationship with: the kidney. As we learned from the other fields of medicine, the body that hosted the kidney was an *emanet* animated through the *jann*, and it existed beyond consciousness, on its own. People did not have a separate relationship with each internal organ. What kind of a loss was the kidney then? How would one make sense of it? How would one mourn it?

Yet, before they could make sense of the lost object, a machine, an apparatus that traditionally invoked feelings of loss of control over the artificial, had taken over their bodies. In hospital rooms while lying next to strangers who welcomed them into their new "dialysis" family, patients began mourning the loss. They were also learning to mourn in new ways, through the ways machines, objects, and institutions had taken over their lives. The history of things, the state, its institutions, the machine, death, the afterlife, the kidney, the *kadavra*, the living donor, suicides, needles, body parts, the organ mafia, political leaders, physicians—all these things they had learned about, *known* of, and kept at a certain distance from their selfhood were now presented to them in an unusual setting, like a history they had to fit into their lives: they had to make these things their own to come to terms with their loss and to find possibilities to exit the machine life.

Life on the machine was not only oppressive because of the routines but also evocative. While patients were trying to liberate themselves from the machine they realized that their suffering had roots in many spheres of life, not only in the machinistic dialysis routines, hospital bureaucracy, or their own poverty but especially in their intimate relationships with their partners and families. Technology had entered their lives only to transform their relationships with the people they felt close to, from their kin to their larger social milieu.

While Zehra was on dialysis, the *dede*, her neighbor in the next bed, began showing her signs that confirmed her own Alevi roots, which led her to react to her family's daily routines and to her faith in the truth of her past, beginning with her relationship to her father. Fidan thought of her head covering and how she had been excluded from public education because of it, just like, she thought, the isolating routines of the machine kept her away from sociality. In the machine, Oğuz saw a possibility, or a new way of fashioning himself, whereas for Hatice, the dialysis machine had taken her away from her daughter because of its routines. Patients confronted the symbolics of the dialysis machine in different ways, either isolating themselves from social life entirely, like Fidan, or believing that a stranger who shared the same destiny could actually be the true relation, like Zehra. While they were feeling overwhelmed by the sudden diagnosis, the invasive dialysis routines, and the new kinship ties with dialysis patients, they would begin hearing legends and myths, and learning about the politics of transplants. This was their entry to a strange new biopolis. It was characterized by a beginning that was marked by the relationship to the dialysis machine.

The machine had long been a metaphor for a grand structure, for control, and for surveillance. The psychoanalyst Victor Tausk studied the relationship between self-integrity and self-control in Vienna using a phenomena of the early 1900s, the "influencing machine," an apparatus imagined, by the patient, to affect the way things truly were; it was an inner world that became visible due to some mental processes that were regarded by that society as abnormal. Tausk was convinced that his patients saw a machine, a device, a system, a network of events that directly controlled their lives.

This appeared generally with a physical surgical intervention to their bodies. One of his patients was so fearful and outraged by what she "realized" that she assumed "they" had "taken over" her body via a machine in Berlin and placed her loved ones under control, all without gaining the notice of others. The influencing machine was what patients saw when they lost the integrity of their bodies and consequently lost the coherence of their sense of being. It showed them a secret hidden structure underlying the surface of events. It was as if they came to realize the truth of their own reality for the first time. The influencing machine was a technology of the self,[1] and like other similar technologies such as sexuality, it operated in the inner world and through metaphors of the artificial, the structure, and the designed. It revealed truth about their present human condition.

The paranoia of "control" and "domination," and the metaphor of "the machine as the grand system," had marked the era of Tausk's diagnosis. Likewise, an unusual feeling had been evoked by the transitional life at the dialysis machine, imposing a change in the relationship between the state, the *jann*, and the body throughout Turkish modernity. This biopolis made the body part of an experiential social contract between the morphing individual and the phantasmagoric world as it slowly became visible from behind the shiny forms and rigid structures of Occidental bureaucracies, neoliberal markets, institutions, and the state. In object relations, in emotion-laden objects, in objects of affect it became more visible. This experience must have united patients' inner selves with realities that used to be at a distance, excluded from their sense of being, "each truer than the one it had enclosed and itself false in relation to the one which encompassed it."[2] The absorption of this kind of reality was a natural part of the human experience, but it was condensed within the forms and norms of the new biopolis in which the metaphors of the machine echoed. Patients must have felt forced to internalize biopolitical objects under such conditions, which in turn must have forced them into a choice about their place in the world, about their selfhoods. Maybe a civil war, a military putsch, a bankruptcy, fears of purgatory, prostitution, or issues related to minority rights were coming to the surface as affects refracted through a new set of senses, a new sensibility.

The change—at once scary, secret, unavoidable—was in part described as a psychotic experience reflected in the eyes of strangers: Zehra had observed the *dede*'s hands, which morphed into hers, *and* physicians' looks that changed color; Oğuz could no longer wash his hands, shave, and recognize his self-reflection in the mirror; Fidan could not explain to herself the causes of her deep depression despite being a religious person grounded in a strong faith in life. These transformations had started soon after they experienced renal failure and were put on dialysis, and then these transformations were amplified with their transplants. The transplant was more than a mere exchange of "parts"; it was like a metamorphosis that manifested itself in the patients' own appearances inside or outside their bodies. As if there were a designed intervention, patients felt they incorporated another realm within themselves entirely, rather than "simply" a kidney from another person, or a mere medical prosthetic in the machine. Through technology, they were internalizing objects of various kinds, and the emerging relationship with them was changing their relationship with life's truth.[3] The modern was no longer a desirable thing, as it used to be, but an invasion in a rather new space, a new life, emerging through structures and technology.

BENİMSEME

Through the years I worked on this material, I tried to understand the elements of this becoming world and with what social mechanisms and psychological processes it eventually would affect our lives. Transplant patients made the biopolis's objects their own, they internalized them and they changed.

In a way, a transplant patient's experience was the opposite of our relationship with nature, a separation that begins in birth and continues to break up in stages, from breastfeeding to the realization of the self through the mirror image. Unlike these infantile separations, the kidney's sociality united people with an *unknown* artificial world invoked throughout the transplant process. Instead of a separation from the ocean of life to a separate ego, this unification initiated by technology was a reversal in the relationship with the courses of life as intended; it was a "physical body" with distant lives, unrelated realities.

To speak of the new life, I have introduced the biopolis, which helps map and spatialize the cultural elements and processes of internalization of the relationship between nature and culture. In the Turkish biopolis, biomedical technologies reinvented rites, utilized old rituals, labeled imported objects, and invented many different techniques to be able to diffuse certain bodies in order to give life to transplant patients, to deal with the dead for the sake of the living. This was no design. On the contrary, most of the physicians or pharmacologists were acting according to their consciences and walking a very fine line that divided the traditions, dignity, and rights from any wrongdoing. Throughout the history of transplants, and in earlier efforts as in anatomy, Turkish physicians had invested much effort in inventing words to be able to speak of death and its place in medicine internally among themselves as well as outside to the patients' families: to make the transplant technologies sound fitting with common-sense death. While patients were hoping for a matching donor, physicians were trying to institutionalize a transitional liminal domain in which the brain-dead donor could exist and transplants could become a practice. This effort was in line with a long tradition of modernity they had borrowed from the West. They had made modernity their own by fitting it to local customs and traditions. As patients were looking forward to completing their vows through gifts, charities, prayers, and other donations, physicians deployed local cultures of rites of passage to turn transplants into a routine practice. To freeze time, to stop the strange impressions, and maybe to allow patients see beyond their incomplete selves, they treated social pressures as a given. The domain they were utilizing was an utterly frail one. Much fear inhabited it. Many people mistrusted physicians; this mistrust had spilled over from the mistrust rooted in the instability of political life, of short-term governments, military interventions, anarchy in the streets, and social inequalities. Patients extended this mistrust to the institutionalization of death for the sake of the living.

In this sense, the biopolis was not a realm where patients and physicians were the two unrelated and separate faces that looked through each other. On the contrary, what was construed, invented, and internalized as a culturally viable object in medicine was made inner, personal, and private in patients' lives. *Benimseme* was as essentially a cultural mechanism as it was a psychological one. Patients learned about their condition by relating to these objects; they began to make sense of their new universe through them, especially through their other half, with which they were locally and culturally reinvented. While patients internalized stories, moralities, norms, and values with the transplant, they became conscious of a transported essence of life, or *jann*, carried in the flesh of the transplanted organs into their bodies. Just like that, the transplanted kidney exceeded its fleshy qualities as an internal organ and became an internal object. In this way, the *jann* inherent in all beings and now internalized as a sociality with the transplant may have made patients feel a shift in reality.

The *jann* of the kidney united the patient with the life-less objects and with all the processes that invented them. Even though it was acquired through processes that resemble normal forms of exchange, the organ was not entirely a commodity, a fetish, stripped of its former owner. It signified the *jann* of someone else inside the patient, if not the spirit of a whole social life. For this reason, the imagined and internalized transplant was a unification with another's life, a human drama staged in the defenseless innerhood going through surgeries and other forms of exchange. *Benimseme* was the most essential quality of subjectivity. Without it, technology could not be personal; without it its emotional affects and turmoil could not be interpreted.

In the first half of the twentieth century writers known as the Frankfurt school spoke of the changing social formations of emotions and affects associated with technology to provide the public with a critique of modernity and capitalism that they had observed in the newborn relationship between the artificial and the self. This affect of modernity expressed itself in identity formation; it was the consequence of an invisible form the artificial had assumed in the language of practices that linked capitalism to all forms of exchange as it linked politics to individual moralities. Similarly, a transplant interrupted the flow of a person's biological history; it was a violation to the "wholeness" of the body. It destabilized one's love for life, for family, and for community. It evoked uncertainty and made uncertainty a permanent predicament of life. It undid the personhood by taking away one's sense of control over one's body such that freedom was believed to be lost in a very literal way. Much more came about in a transplant patient's sense of the self: the biological transformation provoked deeply political and religious associations and transferences.

The human condition of transplant patients taught me how we make our fragmented lives into a meaningful experience through histories of the living and the dead. I learned from them that we become what we are through people and objects that are out of sight, in things murdered, erased, and assimilated by the metaphors of a collective desire to maintain normalcy. These objects, which used to have human life in them in a past sociality, needed names to be reincarnated as biomedical objects. Transplant patients' life histories were crystallizations of these reincarnations. Patients recovered from the loss with a transplant. But as they did so, they began seeing another world more vivid and real than their own that was related to the exception, the abnormality, the taboo, or the excluded. And in time, they began living more in this new reality than in the former one as they embraced this new world and the new self. They changed. To me, their life histories provided the beginnings of psychological platforms marked by the dilated meanings of larger further worlds. I began with the "nearest" to understand what seemed like purely personal, individualized affect and emotion, and followed the cultural traces to the outskirts of the social for this reason. There, marginal worlds that used to be so far, and that came about without their knowledge, attention, or intervention, became their nearest relations. They faced these new relations while they began to believe that inside them something had died and the new thing that would substitute for it had begun to live and take shape through technology. These transplant patients wanted to get back to the "natural" courses of life with the new technological kidney, like seasons attached to the year. Theirs was much less of a cyborgian embrace of the empowered and emancipated person who could fashion and control the machine. It was uncanny. It was "less-than-before," it led to a "second life" or a "reborn life," as patients worded it, in a deconstructed world. It was a human condition in which one had to face the misgivings and realities of a social life in ashes. It was a lonely journey deep into the materializations of the self through the language of the flesh and through the embodiment of all that made up cultural practices, our notion of time, and a feeling for space. It revealed who we were and what we wanted to be, it revealed our human condition and its uncertain futures: it was a shortcut to us, to our becoming literally through the flesh of the Other.

Just like this, biomedical technologies allow us consumers to move through distant realities of life, through bodies of the Other, literally as well as metaphorically, and in this way change the way we relate to life, to nature, and our place in it. They invent epistemic things *unknown* to experience before.[4] They utilize common sense as we let life grow on us.[5] They challenge moral lifeworlds born in distant ethical plateaus.[6] They transform how we view matters of life and death. All these realities come to occupy our inner worlds as parts of a *benimseme,* as we move in millennial economies of capitalism,[7] neither separate from nature nor locked in cultural constructions but through new senses and organs emerging within the fragile universe that occupies our inner lives.

ACKNOWLEDGMENTS

This book started out as a dissertation project. It would not have materialized without the generous support of my advisor at MIT, Michael M. J. Fischer. He encouraged it in all its stages from a virtual project to the book you are reading. His intellectual insights have become essential to my anthropology.

The book owes much to my dissertation committee. Harriet Ritvo taught me how to think like a writer of the English language, and to her I owe much of my affection for writing and for history. Sherry Turkle taught me how to relate external events to inner manifestations and make sense of them. The psychoanalytic process has become an integral part of my thinking thanks to her insights. Joseph Dumit taught me the density and complexity of science and technology studies (STS) scholarship, and he helped the project unfold in the rhythm of this emerging field. Finally João Biehl's passion for social justice was a true inspiration, which transformed the way I see the field, anthropology, and my place in both. His work in Brazil provided me with a lens that helped me see the strengths and vulnerabilities of the culture I was trying to understand.

There are many more people to whom I am greatly in debt. The Friday Seminars at Harvard University's Department of Anthropology were a platform that continuously nourished me intellectually, and the acquaintances I made there have been a part of this book project. Mary-Jo delVeccio and Byron Good's work on subjectivities influenced my thinking from its early days. I thank Maria Pia di Bella, Samer Dewachi, Baber Johansson, Clara Han, Andy Lakoff, and Johan Lindquist. I met Nancy Scheper-Hughes and Lawrence Cohen during these seminars, and started my initial work through their project at Berkeley's Organs Watch. I have kept fond memories of that early work throughout the years. At Harvard, there were other people who became indispensable to the progress of this work. I thank Cemal Kafadar for his interest and faith in this project. I also thank İlay Örs, Chris Dole, and Aykan Erdemir. Their fieldwork in Turkey was contemporary to mine and sharing thoughts and experiences with them made memories of the field more vivid and tangible.

There were friends who followed the changes of this book throughout the years. I thank Adriana Petryna for her own inspiring work and for her sincerity as a scholar and a friend. Simon Schaffer was able to find the right edge to see the material at its best. His friendship was indispensable to this book long before it became an idea. Margaret Lock's scholarship on brain death in Japan and on medical anthropology has helped me to rethink many issues throughout my work on this book. My conversations with Hakan Gürses evoked from early on my interest in critical theory. I thank him for this and for our decades-old friendship.

All of my colleagues, mentors, and friends in the anthropology and history departments and in STS at MIT have been great listeners throughout the years. I thank Deborah Fitzgerald, David Kaiser, Stefan Helmreich, Jean Jackson, Erica James, Evelyn Fox Keller, Philip Khoury, Susan Silbey, Peter Perdue, Rosalind Williams, Charles Weiner, Etienne Benson, Sandy Brown, Candis Callison, Anita Chan, Nathan Greenslit, Rachel Prentice, Meg Hisinger, Hyun Gyun Im, Richa Kumar, Wen-Hua Kuo, David Lusco, Eden Miller, Natasha Myers, Esra Özkan, Anya Zilberstein, Christopher Kelty, Hannah Landecker, Melissa Cefkin, Mazyar Lofalian, Heinrich Schwarz, Regula Burri, Olivia Daste, Susanne Wilkinson, Orkideh Behrouzan, Samer Jabbour, and last but not least Livia Wick, who has been a close friend with a great interest in the unfolding nature of this work. Susanne Koschitz, Duks Koschitz, Sonja Schmidt, Judith Kroell, and Skuli Sigurdson have known my work throughout the years. I am grateful for their friendship.

At Duke University Press, I thank Ken Wissoker for his support from the first day onward, and Tim Elfenbein for his editorial help. The American Research Institute in Turkey helped fund this book in its dissertation stage.

Many people in Turkey, whose names must remain anonymous, uplifted this material with their strength and sensibilities. I owe much to them, especially the dedicated physicians and nurses in Turkey who go through such trying days. Their sincerity in sharing their life histories made this book what it is, because they had the strength to face their misgivings about their everyday decisions, and in this they provided exemplary cases for physicians and health caregivers around the world who shoulder similar burdens.

Working with the photographer Laleper Aytek has been a splendid experience. I feel indebted to her kindness, her talent, and her cooperation.

Finally I thank my parents and my sister for their support. Without the warmth they provided me, I would not have been able to write this book. My aunt Sezan Köksal, who passed away as this book went into production, was a role model to me all of my life and will remain so. Over many years, Lies Cosjin has listened to my fieldwork stories and supported the publication of this book in every way. I have been inspired by her and her late husband Hermann Meijer's commitment to human rights and social justice. And to my husband, Rob Meijers, who almost never lost hope in this work, I owe gratitude. His love nurtured me, the book, and our daughter.

PROLOGUE. THE ACCURATE NATURE OF THINGS

1 I refer here to Lacan's use of the notion of "the real" to speak of things outside the faculty of comprehension. The term does not refer to the state of things or events, but to the strong presence of *unknown* qualities that indicate a turn of events that bridges the imaginary and the symbolic. It is beyond a statement of "fact"—it allows alternative imaginaries to assume truth.

2 Among Alevis, *biz* ("us") is a political category that signifies not only the Alevi identity, but also its difference from Turkey's majority Sunni population. During Alevi *cems*, men and women gather to talk about politics, listen to elders' stories, interpret past events, and talk of daily life concerns, putting into effect the power of *biz* in opposition to *ötekiler*, "the others." Family, *cem*, and community were all signified by the term *biz*. The group enhanced and multiplied individual presence. When Zehra's brother told her that she was "not one of them," he was referring to this kinship and condition of the self in the Alevi community (see Bal, *Alevi-Bektasi köylerinde toplumsal kurumlar*).

3 Turkish scholars believe that Turks' original religion was a form of shamanism that later mingled with Islam. Scholarly comparisons, especially of Alevis, note

commonalities between shamanism and local Muslim saint-worship practices. The roots of this similarity are found in studies of early Turkish texts like the Orhun and Uygur Tablets and the oral tradition of Dede Korkut stories throughout Turkic communities in Asia and Anatolia. See Gökalp, *Türk Töresi*; Bal, *Alevi-Bektasi köylerinde toplumsal kurumlar*; Gökyay, "Dede Korkut hikayelerinde şamanlık izleri."

4 Bal, *Alevi-Bektasi köylerinde toplumsal kurumlar.*

5 Şener, *Alevi törenleri.*

6 According to the political philosopher Hannah Arendt, the spirit of the modern embraces calls for *vita activa*, an ideal combination of speech, politics, and action that is meant to liberate the modern individual (Arendt, *The Human Condition*). Atatürk's reformations aimed to establish a new modern state—"a liberated individual"—from the remnants of Ottoman imperial rule and its subjects. This impulse was welcomed by Alevis at the time, as their communities were traditionally based on egalitarian political decision-making processes and, as a result of centuries of Sufi influence, the balancing of religious orthodoxy against reason for the sake of individual liberties.

7 Mary Douglas (*Purity and Danger*) writes of how culturally salient objects are classified and categorized by means of a cosmological distinction between the clean and the pure on the one hand and the dangerous or contaminating on the other. Zehra perceived the *dede* as a pure object, in this sense, and one that indicates more generally what kinds of objects are incorporated and made one's own when one is trying to hold onto beliefs and values that make one's soul and one's life meaningful. Remaining within the realm of *biz* (us), a basic concept in Alevi culture, Zehra is able to make *dede* her own by seeing physical changes by which he resembles her and thus is hers.

INTRODUCTION. WHAT MAKES THE WORLD OUR OWN

1 Quoted in Löwith, *From Hegel to Nietzsche*, 10.

2 Lacan, *The Psychoses*.

3 Sherry Turkle had posed this problem many years ago in the *Second Self*. Studying our interaction with computers, she tried to understand the effect of computers on our personal development. She was not only interested in how the world would look like as computers became more like people, but what people would become. My question, in a way, follows up on this. In an effort to understand what we are becoming, I look into technologically and politically charged objects, such as allografts, the cadaver body, the suicide or the insane, which operate like linkages that bond worlds to one another. As we experience these objects with an operation, or in vocational practices, we acquire a certain self-knowledge that seems to change us, morph us.

4 See Fischer, "Culture and Cultural Analysis" for an account of the cultural as an active process.

5 On the ways biotechnologies are embraced by physicians and patients alike, see DelVecchio Good, "The Medical Imaginary and the Biotechnical Embrace."

6 On the philology and epistemic history of the *sensus communis*, see Gadamer, *Wahrheit und Methode*.

7 See Geertz, *Interpretation of Cultures*; Fischer, *Iran*; Kleinman, *Patients and Healers in the Context of Culture*.

8 See Fischer, *Anthropological Futures*, chapter 5 for another example of a technological object as a field of object relations.

9 See Gennep, *The Rites of Passage*; Mauss, *The Gift*; Turner, *The Ritual Process*.

10 Scheper-Hughes, "Parts Unknown."

11 Sanal, " 'Robin Hood' of Techno-Turkey."

12 It is biopolitics in a sense that troubled the terms of disciplining and re-educating populations and the nation, and deciding who to let die and who to make live among individual bodies.

13 The divine breath, the *jann*, resides in the person and is "borrowed" and must be returned, like the Maori *hau* made famous in the anthropological literature by Marcel Mauss in *The Gift*.

14 Ritvo, *The Platypus and the Mermaid, and Other Figments of the Classifying Imagination*.

15 Fischer, *Iran*; *Emergent Forms of Life and the Anthropological Voice*; *Anthropological Futures*.

16 Dumit, *Picturing Personhood*.

17 See Turkle, *The Second Self*; *Life on the Screen*; *Evocative Objects*.

18 See Biehl, "Other Life"; "Technology and Affect"; *Vita*.

PART ONE. THE DESIRABLE

1 Here I borrow the word "uncanny" from Freud's book of the same title. According to Freud, the uncanny—in German, *unheimliche*—is an unsettling sensation one experiences as a result of not knowing the source of feelings. The uncanny refers to mysterious events that cannot be known but that at the same time can shed new light on the nature of things if one is given a chance to explore and know them. I also would like to draw attention to Oğuz's expression here: he used the words *tuhaf* and *garib*, meaning literally strange or uncanny. The dialysis machine seems to be the *unknown* external object and the *unknowable* source of suffering in his narrative. Most patients I talked to felt this great distance from it, almost as if they were possessed by it but did not know what it was about.

2 In "Mourning and Melancholia," Freud describes melancholia as the ego-damaging void caused by the loss of a loved person or object. If the void, the loss, is not filled with a substitute object, then the ego is forced into the work of mourning. Oğuz felt the void, the emptiness within, and was shaken by the recurring feeling of being "emptied out," a feeling of loss. In an effort to get rid of the emptiness,

to fill in the void, he drank more than he was supposed to and caused further damage to his body. Unlike the operation of psychological mechanisms—recovery from melancholia by finding a new love, for example—recovery from the physical damage of renal failure works the other way around. The medical aim of getting rid of toxins actually produces a recurring feeling of emptiness for the patients.

3 Oğuz's doctor told me the same thing. In his transplantation unit he had never had a patient whose transplanted kidney lasted more than nine years. A cadaver kidney in particular could last only a few years. By the time it arrived at the hospital, it was already traumatized by hours of storage in ice. Living related transplantations offered better chances, and so he "encouraged" Oğuz that he could expect about nine years of life from his father's kidney.

4 There are many different and personal reasons why women decide to cover their heads. Some do it later in life because of religious devotion or in response to a traumatic experience, and some come from traditional households where all their female family members wear the headscarf. Academic debates on what the form and style of cover symbolize are complex. Political change manifests in different ways and in different transformations of the public sphere, sometimes including the marking of femininity. In this sense covering has been seen as the indication of a boundary, marking the limits of selfhood and the other, inside and outside, the personal and the political. For a further analysis on the politicization of the veil as a symbol of Islam in Turkey in the 1980s, see Göle, *Modern Mahrem*; and for cosmological and anthropological analysis of veiling in Anatolia, see Deleaney, *Tohum ve Toprak*.

5 Brain-death is defined by the death of the brain-stem and other criteria, in which the body can no longer rely on the brain to sustain the body but needs life support.

6 Nancy Scheper-Hughes ("Rotten Trade") has described this kind of medical mobility as "organ tourism," a term she uses specifically to refer to companies that organize travel abroad both for medical and leisure purposes.

7 Here, Fidan refers to the public response to the rapid change of the alphabet. People had to learn the new letters, become accustomed to reading them, and leave the books of yesterday aside. My grandfather, who taught Turkish and Ottoman literature, would complain about this whenever he showed me his collection of books. Much of his library, which he had been assembling since his youth, was in Ottoman, a script that I could not read. As I gazed into his books with what must have looked like a dull expression on my face, my grandfather seemed to become more upset, but he could not put his feelings into words. Sometimes he would complain about the change, but mostly he remained silent, and from his silence I have learned how ordinary people managed under the oppression of transitional regimes. My grandfather was an Oriental, and I had been brought up to live in an imaginary Europe.

8 *Mahrem* is the private, the sphere that is owned by the person. The feeling of retrieving one's privacy shows the patient's ability to reconstruct and repair the world shattered by the loss of the kidney.

9   See Sharp, *Bodies, Commodities, and Biotechnologies,* and Joralemon, "Organ Wars" for brief summaries of the economy of bodies and body parts in the United States. The term "the gift of life" was originally used to describe blood donation, and currently it is also applied to gestational surrogacy (Sharp, *Bodies, Commodities, and Biotechnologies,* 17).

10 Mauss, *The Gift,* 13–14.

11 Ibid., 11–12.

12 Mary Douglas (*Purity and Danger*) argued that boundaries established classifications in social life through purity and danger. The transplanted organ as a gift blurred these boundaries between the self and the other, inside and outside, making the recipient enter a dangerous zone.

13 Fox and Swazey, *Spare Parts,* 40.

14 In 2007 there was an attempt to introduce a close translation of the English "gift of life" as the metaphoric *hayata bağış* to replace the wide colloquial use of the literal phrase *organ bağışı* (organ donation). With a television program and a website launched at CNN-Türk, Münci Kalayoğlu, who had just moved back to Turkey from the United States, and Ata Bozoklar hoped to increase the amount of organ donation by receiving public support.

15 Transplant practices were characterized more by the life-giving quality of organ donation rather than by being an object of exchange or gift despite the semantics of the expression *organ bağışı,* which is formally being related to "sacrificial offering" and to "charitable gift."

16 In her book *Tanrının Yeryüzündeki İşaretleri,* Schimmel, like many others, argues that despite orthodox Islam's denial of the existence of spirits of nature, life energy is everywhere in Anatolian Islam, embedded in religious practices focusing on sacred stones, places, animals, saints, and other objects. I use *Jann* here in the sense of this immanent folk understanding of life-force. It is embedded in all living beings yet different from life. *Jann* carries the ontological characteristics of the objects it occupies but assumes additional powers as well.

17 Ata Bozoklar, "Türkiye'de Organ Nakli" (private presentation, Memorial Hospital, Istanbul, May 17, 2007).

18 Haberal et al., "Transplantation Legislation and Practice in Turkey," 3644–46.

19 History is only complete when its mythical or absent self can be told as a part of the story. The transplant myth embodies many histories beyond the "official" tale provided by physicians and academic writings. According to one source, the first transplant in Turkey was actually done at Istanbul University Hospital right after Christian Bernard performed a heart transplant in South Africa. Turkish doctors who admired Bernard's surgical success thought they could replicate it. The effort fell through and the patient died soon after the operation. This memory of an "untold history" marks transplant knowledge as a process of learning that the success of the practice meant more than just surgery: it required immunosuppressants, dialogue with patients, and careful aftercare.

20 Temizyürek et al., *Basında Transplantasyonun 20 Yılı,* 6.

21 Haberal, "Development of Transplantation in Turkey," 3027.

22 It has since become a hospital, which after twenty-five years performs the highest rate of transplants from brain-dead donors in Turkey.

23 I describe the three legal categories for donation later in this part.

24 Kemal, *Tanyeri Horozları*, 119 (translated by the author).

25 Later on, as Kemal's controversial ideas spread, he was forced to flee to exile in Paris. In 1868 he began the anti-establishment Turkish-language newspaper *Hürriyet* (Liberty) in London. He eventually returned home, only to be exiled again because of the liberal and nationalist ideals in his popular play *Vatan Yahut Silistre* of 1873.

26 Mustafa Kemal started congressional meetings throughout Anatolia to liberate the country from the French, Italian, English, and Greek occupiers. Thus began the Turkish War of Independence (1919–23). In April 1920 the new parliament, the Türkiye Büyük Millet Meclisi (the Turkish Grand National Assembly), was established under Mustafa Kemal's leadership. It abolished the sultanate and forced the last sultan, Mehmed Resad V, into exile.

27 Bozdoğan and Kasaba (*Rethinking Modernity and National Identity in Turkey*, 3) underline the importance of the spirit of youth in the new Turkish republic and its modernization ethos, and they argue that this ethos has penetrated into people's perception of the republic and its future.

28 Güvenç, *Türk Kimliği*, 21–50.

29 See Proctor, *Racial Hygiene* on social Darwinism, anthropology, and eugenics in the early twentieth century.

30 See Güvenç, *Türk Kimliği* for detailed historiographic and ethnographic analysis of the construction of Turkish identity and nation.

31 Foucault, *Ethics*.

32 In an extreme example of this, the origins of Turkishness are symbolically associated with the gray wolf—a mother wolf who cared for a human infant and thereby brought the declining Turkish lineage back to life. In the beginning of the 2000s, the wolf was invoked to represent selfhood and core identity among patriarchal, nationalist, and fascist elements. These political ideologies are further nourished by conspiracy stories such as those in the TV series *Kurtlar Vadisi* (The valley of the wolves, 2003–5) and a 2006 action film spin-off, *Kurtlar Vadisi—Irak* (The valley of the wolves—Iraq), which tell of systematic violence against and exploitation of Muslims, including organ trafficking and the Abu Ghraib torture scandal. *Kurtlar Vadisi* highlights the hegemonic relationship between the United States and Turkey in ways that question notions of sovereignty and freedom in a world of chaos and violence.

33 In a significant symbolic gesture, the DP allowed prayers to be conducted in Arabic again instead of Turkish as soon as it came to power.

34 Under the DP's governance, the Turkish lira was devalued, the IMF began helping with a recovery plan, and immigration from villages to big cities began.

35 On the political history of modern Turkey, see Ahmad, *Bir Kimlik Peşinde Tür-kiye*; Bozdoğan and Kasaba, *Rethinking Modernity and National Identity in Turkey*; White, *Islamist Mobilization in Turkey*.

36 Ideas of individualism and freedom dated all the way back to the Gülhane Hatt-ı Hümayun of 1839 and lived in the collective memory analogous to modernity. With the Gülhane, people had become citizens. Having acquired names and rights, they had become subjects of a bureaucratic enterprise that, they felt, watched and followed them for its own ends. These feelings were expressed by avant-garde poets of the era.

37 George Orwell makes a similar symbolic reference in his famous dystopia *1984*, as his characters experience important revelations in a park under a walnut tree.

38 Hikmet, *Beyond the Walls*, 197.

39 Ibid., 3027.

40 Imuran is an immunosuppressant manufactured by GlaxoSmithKline. Its active ingredient is Azathioprine, which dampens the activity of immune cells.

41 Haberal et al., *Basında Transplantasyonun 20 Yılı*, 9.

42 By the end of that year there were a total of nine stories, their tone shifting from despair to hope as dialysis machines were made available by state insurance soon after the putsch.

43 These experimental efforts, he believed, initiated further study of kidney preservation across the entire field, and reports of renal transplants with cold ischemia times of forty-eight to seventy-two hours began to appear in the literature (Haberal et al.,"Transplantation Legislation and Practice in Turkey," 3644).

44 See Sanal, "'Robin Hood' of Techno-Turkey or Organ Trafficking the State of Ethical Beings"; "Flesh Mine, Bones Yours."

45 The "Ottoman mentality" here refers to contemporary Turkish modernists' perception of a more traditional Ottoman worldview, one that is backward and premodern but at the same time constitutionally and bureaucratically institutionalized.

46 NTV News, interview with Alper Demirbaş, Akdeniz University, May 5, 2007.

47 By 2000, the total number of all cadaver kidney transplantations in Turkey was just over 1,000, whereas in Europe the average transplantation rate is 3,500 per year, and over 95 percent of these are from cadavers. This figure is from an interview with Dr. Eldegez in 2000.

48 These statistics are selected from figures given to me by various doctors during my ethnographic work. Since Ankara and Istanbul maintain completely separate databases, there were no reliable nationwide statistics on organ transplantation. So when people associated with either network talk about the number of transplantations nationwide, they were generally referring only to the quantities indicated by their own databases. The number of patients waiting for kidney transplants is based on the figure repeatedly cited by patients in both Ankara and Istanbul. This was not the "official" number of the people and listings in each hospital, but rather the number of people the patients I spoke to believed were in dialysis

centers nationwide. The problem of statistics requires more extensive work, but I do not have the necessary data to fully engage it at this stage due to inconsistencies on numbers nationwide. In the meantime, however, I would suggest that these numbers can be seen as a part of the efforts by politicians, physicians, and patients themselves to create narratives (including statistical ones) that depict acceptable standards and conditions for treatment.

49 Küçük et al., "Demographic Analysis," 2005.

50 See Pessione et al., "Multivariate Analysis of Donor Risk"; Johnson et al., "Double Renal Allografts"; Perico et al., "Tackling the Shortage of Donor Kidneys."

51 In the United States, the advancement of the medical technology of organ transplantation forced the making and passage of a law on brain-death diagnosis. In Turkey, however, transplantation technology and brain-death diagnosis were legislated simultaneously.

52 Dr. Haberal had a great collection of photographs of Atatürk in his offices. His assistants were fond of this collection; they told me that he even had images of Atatürk no one in the world had seen before. In one meeting room, a portrait of Atatürk was accompanied by one of Atatürk's mother, even larger than Atatürk's, that hung right behind Haberal's desk. The mother figure was festooned all around with reform movement photographs of Atatürk. Two months before I met with Haberal in this room filled with images of Atatürk he had been nominated as a candidate in the upcoming presidential election. "He wants to be the second Atatürk," his assistant told me. Haberal saw his expansion of the definition of kinship for living related donors as protecting people against the corrupting threats of organ trafficking. This "colonization" of the individual body and body politic introduced criminality into the social body. It was this social body that Atatürk had tried in his own time to protect from economic and political colonization.

53 Döşemeci et al., "Brain Death and Donor Management."

54 See ibid., 60.

55 The *hadith* are sayings of Muhammad and his companions. The Sunnah are precedent-setting actions of Muhammad and his companions. *Shar'ia* is the Islamic legal tradition. Karaman, *İslam'ın Işığında Günün Meseleleri*.

56 Karaman, *İslam'ın Işığında Günün Meseleleri*, 792.

57 In Tabakoğlu et al., *Bilgi, Bilim ve İslam II*, the source of this discussion of Islam and medicine, there is a collection of debates and conference notes from a meeting in 1989 of a diverse group of pioneering Turkish scholars of Islam. These scholars argue that the separation between religion and reason in the medical sphere showed itself in the vast number of *ga'yrımüslim* (non-Muslim) doctors who worked to treat Muslim patients in the early ages of Islam. People had trusted their bodies to the Other, the non-Muslim, and in doing so acted upon reason and not religion.

58 The Diyanet's support for organ harvesting from living and dead bodies appears in the transplantation law of 1980 (Haberal, *Doku ve Organ Transplantasyonları*, 11). The legitimation of organ harvesting from cadavers can be found in the principle

that Karaman describes with the statement that "the categorical imperative bends the rules" ("Zaruretler, yasakları kaldırır") (Karaman, "İslam Hukukunda Zaruret Hali," 177). Karaman argues that such practices as the harvesting of corneas and blood transfusions are permissible if the health of the patient can be improved by the body parts of a dead person.

59 Zeydan, "Halat-ud-Darure Fi's- Şeriat'il- İslamiyye," 215.

60 Today, it is almost taken for granted that the Diyanet participates in regulating the donation of organs from cadavers in Turkey. There is not much written on the basic rights of the person that underlie the implementation of this new form of cannibalism. Even though scholars know where the analogy comes from, they do not articulate it to the public as such, they do not speak of cannibalism as analogous to organ transplantations. And past internal debates among Islamic legal scholars on the value of cadavers for medical purposes do not enter into popular discourse. The *fatwa*, a speech act of the Ministry of Health, serves as a supporting narrative in media efforts to raise consciousness about organ donation. These declarations describe the legitimization of cadaveric organ harvesting in terms of an *insanî* (humane) act. But they do not reflect on the nature of *insan* (the human) or its qualities in these declarations. Organ donation is depicted as an altruistic action, rather than in the terms of *zaruret* (emergency) by which cannibalism is legitimized. The respective institutional natures of Islamic scholars and medical experts seem close to each other at this point, especially in the way they internalize technology while creating a "special" logic for its implementation. When both groups engage the public, they speak of the quality of *insan* and its merits; they do not reflect on their internal debates. *İnsan* is the common point of agreement.

61 Maybe because of its uncanny reference to cannibalism, this technical analogy is not referred to in the debates on Islam and organ donation. Instead, organ donation is represented by the Ministry of Health and the media as an act of altruism and humanity.

62 Örnek Buken, "Organ Aktarımlarında Beyin Ölümünün Tıbbi, felsefi ve Teolojik Yönleri," 84.

63 Wijdicks, "Brain Death Worldwide."

64 Gökmenoğlu, *İslâm'da Şahsiyet Hakları.*

65 Ibid., 102–7.

66 Erkol et al., "Initiation of Bone and Amnion Banking in Turkey," 169–72.

67 While the import of allograft from Eastern European countries was becoming a central concern for Ahmed's company, for transplants, Bulgaria was seen as an emerging organ market in the Balkans to pursue such operations—especially since Turkish authorities have exposed Dr. S. and made Turkey a difficult place for illegal transplantations.

68 There is a difference between tissue rejection and organ rejection. When the body's immune system rejects a kidney, for example, the rejection shows up in renal function tests. The only sign of allograft rejection, however, is an infection

around the bone tissue. Orthopedists say that the causes of such infections are impossible to determine.

69 To be precise this was an increase from 255,950 billion TL to 3,674,262 TL.

70 See Başoğlu Hülya, *Uluslararası Rekabet Stratejileri* for the first Turkish Industrialists' and Businessmen Association (TÜSİAD) report on biotechnology.

71 Bora, "Turgut Özal."

72 Yayla, "Özal."

73 Here I refer to Michael Fischer's idea of the "ethical plateau" (*Emergent Forms of Life and the Anthropological Voice*), which is an ethnographic device to locate the different voices represented in bioethical debates. By using it, the anthropologist not only situates himself among other debates that run parallel but also acknowledges the collective ground upon which each single plateau rises and faces the others.

74 In *Homo Sacer* Agamben distinguishes "bare life" from "political existence," as defined by Arendt's *vita activa* of speech, politics, and action. Bare life is real life that exists and operates beyond language and consists of practices that categorize humans as less than *zoë*, or less than profane. It is the realm described by the word "shock," a world of values that we prefer not to know, a world in which categorically there should be no human life, a world beyond the distinctions of the sacred and the profane.

75 See Kemal, *Yer Demir, Gök Bakır* for a picturesque illustration of people's spirit in the region.

76 Sanal, "'Robin Hood' of Techno-Turkey or Organ Trafficking the State of Ethical Beings."

77 *Arena*, February 2000, Channel D, Turkey.

78 I have heard of only male sellers in this context, unlike those female sellers in India we know of from Cohen's work "'Where it hurts.'"

79 "Böbreği satan Filistinli, alan İsrailli, takan Türk," *Vatan*, May 17, 2007.

80 I was stunned by the media emphasis on the threat of looters and the organ mafia during the weeks after the earthquake in Istanbul. In addition, each time I talked about my work, I was reminded of the earthquake by those who believed that looters stole organs from dying people who were trapped and awaiting rescue under the ruins of their own homes.

81 Freud (*Jokes and Their Relation to the Unconscious*) writes that the popular and literary references people make in jokes reveal the legitimacy of particular economies and power relations. In early twentieth-century Vienna, he observed that people joked about their vocations in order to situate themselves within a public rhetoric that displayed the social status of both the vocation and the person's ethnic and religious affiliation.

82 Here I specifically mean the German word *Notstand*—emergency, necessity—a condition that can become the core element upon which a whole institutional structure is founded. The genealogy of the "state of exception" is traced in Agam-

ben, *State of Exception*, along with its relation of exception to the execution of sovereign power.

PART TWO. THE IMPOSSIBLE

1 One of the caretakers of Eyüb Sultan's tomb referred to it as "the City of the Dead" when we spoke, and he told me that it has been called this for centuries. The name is also used by Recep Akakuş, who was the mufti of Eyüb in the 1970s, in his writing (Akakuş, *Eyyüb Sultan*).

2 El-Fatiha is the first verse in the Quran, and is an opening verse for prayers. It is praised for its many qualities, and in popular books on prayers, such as Yusuf Tavaslı's book *Tam Dua Kitabı* (The complete book of prayers), it is recommended for its healing qualities and for protection against the evil eye, witchcraft, illness, and other afflictions.

3 While I was sitting in the mosque of Eyüb Sultan—right across from his tomb—and watching men and women praying, I noticed that every few minutes a cell phone would ring and its owner would run out anxiously. The phone belonging to a man who was sitting close to me rang, and he answered it quietly without leaving the mosque. "I was at the hospital," he said. "Now I am at Eyüb Sultan. When I am done here, I will get back to the hospital." Like most people around us, except for the tourists, he was shuttling between the hospital and the tomb of Eyüb, hoping his prayers would be received by God through the saint's powerful memory embedded in his corpse.

4 According to the legend, one time when the daughter of a Byzantine king became very ill, she was brought to Eyüb's grave to drink the sacred water. She was healed at once. The Byzantines cared for the tomb and the sacred water despite its belonging to a Muslim warrior. When the crusaders invaded Constantinople in 1204 CE, they destroyed the tomb along with many churches (Akakuş, *Eyyüb Sultan*, 54).

5 *Hodja* (spelled *Hoca* in Turkish) is an honorific for the learned.

6 Dabbet-ül Arz is mentioned in the Qur'an twice, but without these mythical characteristics. It is one of the indicators of the Day of Judgment. The medical writer Özkalıpçı has compared the grotesque image of this creature with organ transplantation in her essay "Bir Transplantasyon hayali olarak Dabbet-ül Arz," ironically commenting on where myths and human fantasy lead.

7 I use a translated version (*English Translation of al-Qur'an al-Kerim*, 2007) of the Arabic Qur'an into English via Turkish to bring the reader close to the feelings evoked in the Turkish translation, close to the Turkish interpretation of the Qur'an. The translator, Niyazi Kahveci, thinks that the translation is closer to the Turkish reading; it is a plain and literal one, which he prepared after he had studied the English versions as well as the Arabic original.

8 Smith and Haddad, *The Islamic Understanding of Death and Resurrection*.

9 "The Hour" is another term for Kıyamet (Qur'an 31:34, 74:47).

10 Smith and Haddad, *The Islamic Understanding of Death and Resurrection*, 5.

11 The only exceptions to this mirror-image re-creation are resurrected martyrs, whose bodies were destroyed in war and who are believed to be re-created in a supremely beautiful image.

12 Dr. Osman, a Turkish brain surgeon whom I met at Harvard prior to my fieldwork, told me the tragic story of the pool of the dead. Its image has haunted me since then. As my fieldwork unfolded in unexpected ways, and I decided to write on death and spaces of death and dying, his narrative echoed in my mind.

13 The situation in nineteenth-century England was similar. Ruth Richardson, in her book *Death, Dissection and the Destitute*, describes the implementation of the Body Act of 1832 in England to protect the corpses of the bourgeoisie from grave robbers. The situation in England was so extreme that the rich paid great sums of money to have their graves secured with heavy stones so that their bodies could not be stolen.

14 Ibid.

15 Kahya, "Bizde disseksiyon."

16 Gökalp, *Türk Töresi*.

17 Richardson, *Death, Dissection and the Destitute*.

18 The calendar was reformed in 1923 as part of the progressive ascension to modernity, placing Turkey in the same time scale as the West.

19 Disabled people, like the mentally ill, may be abandoned if no one can take care of them. The biography of this woman resembles that of Mehmed's sister. This resemblance is enhanced by the fact that in an enclosed community such as a village or a religious congregation, the relationships among men and women include a feeling of extended kinship: they become sisters and brothers, even if they are not biologically related. To me the overlapping biographies of these two people with the same disability—muteness—show the formation of their ties in their social abandonment. For this reason, I thought of this woman as Mehmed's sister, not his real biological sister, but his new sister in abandonment and death.

20 Unat, *Dünya'da ve Türkiye'de 1850 yılından sonra Tıp Dallarındaki İlerlemelerin Tarihi*.

21 Historically, however, there are also examples of torturous treatments for mental illness in various shrines of Anatolia, along with music and water therapies (ibid., 381). The first *bimarhane* was established by Sultan Beyazit II in Edirne. Evliya Çelebi, the famous Ottoman travel writer, describes this *bimarhane* as a place where the ill received food and healing, including music therapy. After the conquest of Istanbul, Sultan Mehmed founded the second *bimarhane* in Istanbul. In the nineteenth century, after Tanzimat, foreign doctors were invited to these *bimarhanes* for scholarly studies (ibid., 379).

22 The shadow theater is a show in which the shadows of two-dimensional puppets are cast upon a screen. It is believed to have been brought to Turkey by Arabs who were influenced by Indonesian puppet traditions.

23 This is also a common narrative pattern found in jokes about the insane.

24 See the resonances of "spaces of exclusion" in Taussig's "spaces of death" (*Shamanism, Colonialism, and the Wild Man*), and Biehl's work on social zones of abandonment (*Vita*), both ethnographies on Latin America specifically defining the territories of how inequalities and social violence mold the geographic space, separating people in the name of domination and colonialism. Petryna's work in Ukraine (*Life Exposed*) also speaks of Chernobyl as a space of exclusion that invents a new understanding of citizenship.

25 The anatomists in particular took great pride in showing me their collection of anatomy atlases. They recounted how Germans had been the initiators, followed by the French, and that these days *Gray's Atlas of Anatomy* and the Visible Human Project made the Americans the leaders in the field.

26 In the contemporary medical education system in Turkey, doctors are required to take a proficiency exam right after their six-year medical education. The exam is difficult and ranks each medical discipline according to its "value." Surgery departments are the hardest to get into, and science- and research-oriented disciplines rank the lowest. This ranking by specialty is linked to the income a new doctor can expect upon graduation. Plastic surgery and cardiac surgery are the highest ranking professions, whereas public health, anatomy, and physiology rank very low. This businesslike organization of medical practice becomes in the end the measure of individual doctors' intelligence and talent.

27 Dr. Vural believes that he was the first to practice acupuncture in Turkey. As a young doctor in the 1970s, he went to Germany and Austria to get a degree in acupuncture and he has been practicing it in a private clinic since then. According to him, there is nothing "mysterious" about acupuncture, a long-standing point of ridicule from other doctors. The body is filled with an electrical wiring system that modern medicine calls the nervous system. Acupuncture intervenes in this system and stimulates the brain functions, normalizing the organism. When the new administration came to power, it allowed Dr. Vural to open the first acupuncture unit in the hospital. It is located just inside the anatomy labs. "This way, acupuncture is a part of the medical curriculum now. We also have research plans to use cadavers to understand the nervous system," he told me.

28 Even though this life is open to change and debate and thus is profane, the afterlife promises stability. Texts describing heaven and hell are detailed and clear. There is no dispute about their reality, since if one doubted the Qur'an one would no longer be considered a Muslim. Hence the written words describing the stages of life and afterlife have the power of timeless truth. The authority of these words on the reality of the afterlife remains unchanged, regardless of changes in morality and religious practice in this life that are open to interpretation.

29 The creation of the new life for the abandoned in the anatomy lab, the transitional phase, can be seen as the product of the anatomists' confrontation with the taboos around death, abandonment, and the ritualistic character of dissection. The soul, trapped in the lab, has to be rendered as once again social in order to sustain the

order of life and death. With the transitional phase, the anatomists invent an acceptable form of time—the non-time of liminality that Turner describes (*The Ritual Process*)—and labor and personhood for the decaying bodies of the abandoned that make it possible for them to procure cadavers, talk to patients' relatives, and relate dissection to medical students and themselves. It is thus the rejection of any transitional phase that creates grounds for the invention of this stage for the mentally ill to become persons again, but only after death. These traumatic conditions for dissection give anthropologists the opportunity to see the purposes for which personhood and labor are invented and how reburial serves as a space in which the construction of the human is explored. At the same time, anatomists struggle constantly to feel like humans themselves while practicing this traumatizing vocation.

30 Lacan (*Écrits*) writes of the first stage in the formation of the self, the "I," as the identification of the other, which he calls the *mirror stage*. The child recognizes his body through recognition of his image in the mirror or in the form of another person. This identification takes place when the subject takes on a self-image. This self-image is registered in what Lacan calls the *imaginary*. Ego formation is an attempt to organize the body and the self in a coherent order. An alienating identification based on the lack of completeness of the body and its environment takes place in ego formation. If the mirror stage is a condition of continuously alienating identification with the Other from which the imaginary is created, then the anatomist's encounter with Mehmed's body image in the mirror on the wall and the dark spots on the surface of the mirror—Mehmed's soul—shows how the passage of the soul of the dissected appears incomplete in the lab. The lab becomes a liminal space; unable to maintain the boundaries between this and other worlds, it invites those other worlds into the shaping of its practices. It becomes a traumatic space where anxiety is nourished by the displacement of the body and the soul, making dissection an undesirable ritual.

31 Printing presses were first set up by Jewish refugees from Spain in Istanbul in 1493, and then in Salonika in 1512. They printed Bibles and prayer books, secular works, and multilingual concordances (Hill, *Hebraica*). But the first Muslim presses were not established until the 1720s by İbrahim Müteferrika (Fischer and Abedi, *Debating Muslims*), who is known as the father of the Ottoman printing press for this reason.

32 Kazancıgil, *XIX. Yüzyılda Osmanlı İmparatorluğunda Anatomi*.

33 Ibid., 17–18.

34 Ibid., 14.

35 In Corbin, *The Man of Light in Iranian Sufism*, one can find all the elements of Sufism and their symbolics discussed as a part of history of sufi traditions and their embodiment in different prophets.

36 İskender, *Cangüncem* (the author's translation).

37 Karaman, *İslam'ın Işığında Günün Meseleleri*; Gökmenoğlu, *İslâm'da Şahsiyet Hakları*.

38 Şehirli et al., "Attitudes of Turkish Anatomists"; Bilgel et al., "Public Attitudes toward Organ Donation."

39 Daar, "The Evolution of Organ Transplantation in the Middle East."

40 İskender, *Cangüncem* (the author's translation).

41 This inheritance procedure is a part of Islamic law and has no binding status in contemporary Turkish law. However, all Turkish state law is informed by Islamic law, and the latter still shapes the rituals and routines that are followed after death. See Keskioglu, *Fıkıh Tarihi ve İslâm Hukuku*, 254–55.

42 Gökmenoğlu, *İslâm'da Şahsiyet Hakları*.

43 Ibid., 56–59, 65–80.

44 Arkun, *Intiharın Psikodinamikleri*.

45 Karaman, *İslam'ın Işığında Günün Meseleleri*. The interpretation of these texts follows methods such as comparison, analogy, categorical imperative, and generalization. The role of these texts is to protect the person.

46 Karaman refers to Muslim Egyptian scientist Resit Rıza, who declared autopsy *caiz* (legitimate) in 1907. Anatomical dissection was permitted by the Ottomans during Tanzimat (1839–76) under a law similar to England's Body Act of 1832 (Karaman, *İslam'ın Işığında Günün Meseleleri*, 792).

47 Gennep, *The Rites of Passage*.

48 Taussig, *Shamanism, Colonialism, and the Wild Man*.

49 Freud, *The Uncanny*, 132.

50 Turner, *The Ritual Process*.

51 The Qur'anic verse quoted in the epigraph is widely cited by transplant doctors when they speak of the virtues of cadaveric donation. It is also referred to by two transplant doctors from Haydarpaşa Numune Hospital in a paper they wrote on transplant ethics to point to Islam's positive attitude toward preserving life. Titiz et al., *Renal Transplantasyona Pratik Yaklaşım*.

52 See Taşdemir and Genç, "Çıldırtan Ayrılık."

53 See Altaylı, "Teke Tek."

54 In the previous ten years only 1,212 people had filled out the organ donation cards at Istanbul University's transplantation unit. Within three months of the praise-filled broadcasts about Ebru Esler's gift of life to six strangers, 4,615 people had asked for donation forms. See "Gündem: Ebru Olayından Sonra Organ Bağışı Arttı"; "Gündem: Organ Bağışında Büyük Artış Var."

55 One of the elements that mobilized the media to this dramatic pro-transplantation blitz—with the support of the Ministry of Health—was the death of a young newspaper reporter named Nurcan Çakıroğlu, who died while waiting to receive a liver transplant. "Gündem: Organ Bağışında Büyük Artış Var."

56 Coşkun, "Gündem."

57 Ibid.

58 Ibid.

59 "Gündem: Arkadaşın Ortak Kaderi."

60 The place tragedy occupies in modern life is transformative for subjectivities. In Ebru's case, with tragedy giving birth to legend, the form is made sublime, and the violent Dionysian and static Apollonian forms of becoming—as Nietzsche describes in *The Birth of Tragedy*—are replaced with modern media and transplant teams with human creators, molding the body through technologies, replacing mythic Gods.

61 There is an inverse relationship between Islam and suicide. According to Lester, in "Suicide and Islam," the Muslim populations in some provinces of India are exceptions to this phenomenon.

62 Ibid.

63 Bonnafous stressed that it was Muslims who suffered most from what Durkheim had theorized as anomic suicide caused by rapid social change in which expectations about the relation between past and future were radically upset. See Arkun, *İntiharın Psikodinamikleri*, 103. There was a higher than usual female suicide rate in the 1920s and 1930s, but it was not higher than that for men. This study was corrected later because it failed to account for the male-female ratio of the population during those years.

64 Bağlı and Sever, "Female and Male Suicides in Batman, Turkey."

65 Arkun, *İntiharın Psikodinamikleri*.

66 Yılmaz, "Victims, Villains and Guardian Angels: Batman Suicide Stories."

67 Arkun, *İntiharın Psikodinamikleri*, 102. The republic declared its liberation from the Ottoman Empire in 1923. In 1924, Hilafet, the institution through which the Ottomans had enforced *shar'ia* law in its Muslim territories, was banned; in 1925, all denominations were banned.

68 A young Turkish woman told me the story of her grandmother, who said she felt naked on the day all women were forced to put their veils, scarves, and other coverings away and dress in dresses, skirts, and jackets. As the wife of the governor, she was ordered to open the dance floor at a ball with her husband. It was styled after European balls—she had to dress in a long dress and dance the waltz. She told her granddaughter it was the greatest embarrassment of her life.

69 Arkun, *İntiharın Psikodinamikleri*, 102–3.

70 Ibid., 98.

71 Karaman, *İslâm'da Şahsiyet Hakları*. The Muslim burial ritual projects the limits of this world and the infinity of cycles, purity and impurity, one's place in the world and in the afterlife. The burial ritual, which sustains the life of the Muslim's soul until the Day of Judgment arrives, cannot accommodate suicide. Because they have taken away what is not theirs, people who have committed suicide are excluded from the order, cleanliness, and purity to which an observant Muslim belongs. As with non-Muslims, there could be no traditional burial for those who have committed suicide, although this is a condition that has changed over the

years, as we have seen. In *İntiharın Psikodinamikleri*, Arkun refers to the *fıkh* that specifically prohibits saying the burial prayer for suicides—one is allowed to pray for the salvation of a man condemned to death but not for one who has interfered with the life cycle ordained by God.

72 Arkun, *İntiharın Psikodinamikleri*.

73 Ibid., 107.

74 Aydın, "Suicide Has Become Fate," quoted in Yılmaz, "Victims, Villains and Guardian Angels."

75 Şen, "The Truth Behind the Suicides," quoted in Yılmaz, "Victims, Villains and Guardian Angels."

76 Kardeşoğlu, "Batman, The City Where Hope Dies," quoted in Yılmaz, "Victims, Villains and Guardian Angels."

77 To probe the rising suicide rate in Batman and the related national news coverage in 2000, four researchers from the Institute of Family Research, who had been invited by the governorship of Batman Province, conducted an assessment inquiry and visited concerned public authorities in Batman. They studied official data on reported suicides and suicide attempts occurring from January 1, 1995, through December 10, 2000, from the Batman police archives, along with the records of the Command of the Provincial Gendarme and other administrative sources outside the municipal hub of Batman. The rates of suicide had increased dramatically.

78 Bağlı and Sever, "Female and Male Suicides in Batman, Turkey."

79 See Çakır, *Derin Hizbullah* for his study on Islam and violence in Turkey. Drawing on the experience of other countries such as Egypt and Algeria and the complicated and deep structures involved in political violence in Turkey, Çakır writes on the views and actions of Hizboullah in Turkey.

80 Çetin, "Suicide Attempts and Self-Image Among Turkish Adolescents."

81 Sever and Erkan, "The Dark Faces of Poverty, Patriarchal Oppression, and Social Change."

82 Ibid.

83 These cases pose questions different from the suicide cases in Istanbul that are directly linked to organ transplantation. These other cases are important because they open up a discourse of the commodification of the female body and suicide as drama and exception.

84 In a talk at Harvard, Pamuk revealed his impressions of Batman and how he wrote *Kar*, translated into English as *Snow*.

85 Yılmaz, "Victims, Villains and Guardian Angels," 73.

86 Press release of Mehmet Nuri Yılmaz, the President of the Presidency of Religious Affairs, October 5, 2000. Available at http://www.byegm.gov.tr/.

87 This relationship, inhered in the body-soul dualism of all three major monotheist world religions, seemed to define the core of any property-commodity relationship. William James had famously asked of bodily ownership whether our bodies were simply ours, or if they were us. The question underlined the duality inherent both in the monotheist religions' idea of the "human" torn between body and the

soul and the Cartesian science based on this duality; both were epistemic conditions rooted in ownership.

88 Özkalıpçı, "Bir Transplantasyon hayali olarak Dabbet-ül Arz."

89 Marc Quinn is a contemporary British sculptor. "His reputation still hangs around his 1991 Blood Head, the frozen cast of his own head which acquired an abstract afterlife consistent with its original concept when the freezer at its owner Charles Saatchi's home was accidentally unplugged and the head melted into a pool of blood" (Steward, "Waxing Lyrical on the Fragile Body").

90 On the place of the aesthetic in the experience and perception of life, see Cassirer, *Rousseau, Kant, Goethe*. According to Cassirer, aesthetic perception is much richer than sense perception and is brought about by the nature of artistic production. The artist unites both worlds, enriching the experience of the object. "In the work of the artists these possibilities become actualities; they are brought into the open and take on a definite shape" (ibid., 145).

91 The Diyanet's *İlmihal*, a two-volume description of authorized Islamic practice in Turkey, includes a ten-page section on sacrifice and the acceptable techniques for sacrificial rituals. *İlmihal* locates the roots of sacrifice in Adam's gift of his two sons to God as sacrificial objects (Qur'an 5:27). The text makes a distinction in the way sacrificial objects are incorporated into religious practice in Islam, Judaism, and Christianity, arguing that in Christianity sacrifice attained a totally new meaning with Jesus's crucifixion and self-sacrifice became an altruistic act. See *İlmihal II*, 2–11.

92 Sacrifice is intertwined with many other practices. For example, if an adult puts on perfume, henna, or hair gel during the Hac, it is a violation of bodily purity at a key time, and he or she would then be obliged to sacrifice an animal to atone for this sin (Erginer, *Kurban*, 142–51).

93 İlyas is Elias or Elijah in the English version of the Greek and Hebrew respectively.

94 See Erginer, *Kurban*. In the case of organ transplantations, patients who have renal failure make vows to perform a sacrifice if they receive a kidney, and after they have the transplantation the first thing their loved ones do is sacrifice whatever animal they can afford to show their gratitude to God. After a transplant operation, I was talking to Hatice, a patient who received a kidney from her sister. She was in bed recovering. With a big smile on her face, the first thing she told me was the good news she had just gotten: her husband had sacrificed a sheep because their prayers had been answered.

95 Eliade, *The Myth of the Eternal Return*.

96 Durkheim, *The Elementary Forms of Religious Life*; Hubert and Mauss, *Sacrifice*. For an analysis of such dialogues in the Zoroastrian *yasna* liturgy, an analogue of the ancient Vedic sacrifices, *yagna*, see Fischer, *Mute Dreams, Blind Owls and Dispersed Knowledges*.

97 Hubert and Mauss, *Sacrifice*, 20–23.

98 Ibid., 37.

99 Conversely, "If the victim was associated with evil, then the destruction and elimination involved the whole body and not only certain parts of it. In the Hebrew
'olah, as in the Greek *holocaust*, the victim was burned in its entirety upon the
altar or within the sacred place, without anything being taken away from it," so
that its impurity was totally destroyed (ibid., 38).

100 I did not find any publication or official declaration from the Diyanet on this
specific justification of the use of suicides for transplants, nor anything against
it. Physicians have always acted with caution and with the Diyanet's support on
these matters. Since the matter was such a public issue, I was confident this senior
physician's statement supported others and that they acted with the Diyanet's
consent and "good intentions," aimed at the redemption of the suicides.

101 For more on how sura 5 of the Qur'an has been used to explain a religious approach to transplantation, see Titiz, *Renal Transplantasyona Pratik Yaklaşım*, 76.

102 See the headlines in *Posta* from February 13, 2002.

103 Agamben, *Homo Sacer*.

104 See Arkun, *İntiharın Psikodinamikleri*, 1.

105 The question of whether Euripides' *Medea* is really about sacrifice is discussed by
Aelius Theon of Alexandria in his work *Progymnasmata*; Theon concluded that
Medea's actions were in fact homicide, not a sacrifice. In Erginer's *Kurban* with
reference to Eliade's *Mitlerin Özellikleri*.

106 Kalyoncu, *Kurban*, summarized from the play, 12–15.

107 Gennep, *The Rites of Passage*.

CONCLUSION. NEW LIFE

1 See Foucault, *Ethics*.

2 Lévi-Strauss, *Tristes Tropique*, 412.

3 See more on how technology changes identity in Turkle (*The Second Self; Life on
the Screen*), where she speaks of the invention of a second self as a result of our
newly emerging relationship with computers. In her analysis, Turkle speaks of
how personhood changes, how people become like machines as they incorporate
them more and more into their lives.

4 See Rheinberger, *Toward a History of Epistemic Things*; Landecker, *Culturing Life*;
Knorr-Cetina, *Epistemic Cultures*; Turkle, *Life on the Screen*.

5 See Fischer and Abedi, *Debating Muslims*; Geertz, "Common Sense as a Cultural
System"; Kleinman, *Patients and Healers in the Context of Culture*.

6 Fischer, *Emergent Forms of Life*.

7 See Comaroff and Comaroff, *Millennial Capitalism and the Culture of Neoliberal-
ism*; Das, *Remaking a World*; Sunder-Rajan, *Biocapital*; Cohen, "Where It Hurts";
Lock, *Twice Dead*; Lock and Crowley-Matoka, "Organ Transplantation in a Glob-
alized World"; Peterson, "HIV/AIDS and Democracy in Nigeria"; Petryna, *Life
Exposed*; Petryna, Lakoff, and Kleinman, *Global Pharmaceuticals*; Biehl, *Vita*;
Biehl, *The Will to Live*.

Agamben, Giorgio. *Homo Sacer: Sovereign Power and Bare Life*. Stanford, Calif.: Stanford University Press, 1998.

——. *State of Exception*. Chicago: University of Chicago Press, 2005.

Ahmad, Feroz. *Bir Kimlik Peşinde Türkiye*. İstanbul: İstanbul Bilgi Universitesi Yayınları, 2007.

Akakuş, Recep. *Eyyüb Sultan ve mukaddes emanetler.* İstanbul: Eyüp Sultan Dini Hizmetler Derneği, 1973.

Altaylı, F. "Teke Tek: Ebruya Değil Aileye Bakın." *Hürriyet,* November 13, 1997.

Anar, İhsan Oktay. *Puslu kıtalar atlası*. İstanbul: İletişim, 2002.

Arendt, Hannah. *The Human Condition*. Chicago: University of Chicago Press, 1998. First published in 1958.

Arkun, Nezahat. *İntiharın Psikodinamikleri*. İstanbul: Baha Matbaası, 1963.

Aydın, G. "Suicide Has Become Fate." *Hürriyet,* October 27, 2000.

Bağlı, M., and A. Sever. "Female and Male Suicides in Batman, Turkey: Poverty, Social Change, Patriarchal Oppression and Gender Links." *Women's Health and Urban Life: An International and Interdisciplinary Journal* 2, no. 1 (2003): 60–84.

Bal, Hüseyin. *Alevi-Bektaşi köylerinde toplumsal kurumlar: Burdur ve Isparta'nın iki Alevi köyünde yapılmış köy araştırması.* İstanbul: Ant Yayınları, 1997.

Başoğlu Hülya, Çetindamar Dilek. *Uluslararası rekabet Stratejileri: Türkiyede Biyoteknoloji İşbirlikleri.* TÜSİAD Rekabet Stratejileri Dizisi-9. TÜSİAD-T/2006/06–421: 128.

Benjamin, Walter. *Moscow Diary.* Ed. Gary Smith. Trans. Richard Sieburth. Cambridge, Mass.: Harvard University Press, 1986. First published in 1927.

Bergson, Henri. *Introduction to Metaphysics.* Indianapolis: Hackett Publishing, 1999. First published in 1912.

Biehl, João. "Biotechnology and the New Politics of Life and Death in Brazil: The AIDS Model." *Princeton Journal* 5 (2002): 59–74.

————. "Other Life: AIDS, Biopolitics and Subjectivity in Brazil's Zones of Social Abandonment." Ph.D. diss., University of California, Berkeley, 1999.

————. "Technology and Affect: HIV-AIDS Testing in Brazil." With Denise Countiho and Ana Luzia Outerio. *Culture, Medicine and Psychiatry* 25, no. 1 (2001): 87–129.

————. *Vita: Life in a Zone of Social Abandonment.* Berkeley: University of California Press, 2005.

————. *The Will to Live: AIDS Therapies and the Politics of Survival.* Princeton, N.J.: Princeton University Press, 2007.

Bilgel, H., N. Bilgel, N. Okan, S. Kılıçturgay, Y. Özen, and N. Korun. "Public Attitudes toward Organ Donation: A Survey in a Turkish Community." *Transplant International* 4 (1991): 243–45.

"Böbreği satan Filistinli, alan İsrailli, takan Türk." *Vatan,* May 17, 2007.

Bora, T. "Turgut Özal." In *Modern Türkiyede Siyasi Düşünce,* vol. 7, *Liberalizm,* 592. İstanbul: İletişim, 2005.

Bozdoğan, Sibel, and Reşat Kasaba, eds. *Rethinking Modernity and National Identity in Turkey.* Seattle: University of Washington Press, 1997.

Çakır, Ruşen. *Derin Hizbullah: İslamcı Şiddetin Geleceği.* İstanbul: Metis, 2001.

Cassirer, Ernst. *The Philosophy of the Enlightenment.* Boston: Beacon Press, 1955.

————. *Rousseau, Kant, Goethe: Two Essays.* Trans. James Gutmann, Paul Oskar Kristeller, and John Herman Randall Jr. Princeton, N.J.: Princeton University Press, 1945.

Çelik, Zeynep. *The Remaking of İstanbul: Portrait of an Ottoman City in the Nineteenth Century.* Berkeley: University of California Press, 1993.

Çetin, Füsun Çuhadaroğlu. "Suicide Attempts and Self-Image Among Turkish Adolescents." *Journal of Youth and Adolescence* 30, no. 5 (2001):641–51.

Çetingüleç, M. "Bad Examples." *Sabah,* January 19, 2001.

Cogito. "Biz Nerede Hata Yaptık?" In *Deprem Özel Sayısı.* Istanbul: YKY, 1999, 290–337.

Cohen, Lawrence. "Operability, Bioavailability and Exception." Medical Anthropology and Cultural Psychiatry Seminar Series. Department of Anthropology, Harvard University, Cambridge, May 2003.

————."'Where It Hurts': Bioethics and Beyond." *Daedalus* 128, no. 4 (1999): 143–49.

Comaroff, Jean, and John L. Comaroff, eds. *Millennial Capitalism and the Culture of Neoliberalism*. Durham, N.C.: Duke University Press, 2001.

Conrad, Joseph. *Heart of Darkness*. New York: Penguin Books, 1999.

Corbin, Henry. *The Man of Light in Iranian Sufism*. Boulder, Colo.: Shambhala, 1978.

Coşkun, N. "Gündem: Can Kardeşler." *Hürriyet*, December 6, 1997.

Çubukçu, Agah. 1989. *Türk—İslam Düşünürleri*. Seri 24, no. 8. Ankara: Türk Tarih Kurumu Basınevi.

Daar, A. S. "The Evolution of Organ Transplantation in the Middle East." *Transplant Proceedings* 31 (1999): 1070–71.

Das, Veena. *Remaking a World: Violence, Social Suffering and Recovery*. Berkeley: University of California Press, 2001.

Davis, Mike. *Ecology of Fear: Los Angeles and the Imagination of Disaster*. New York: Vintage, 1999.

Deleaney, Carol. *Tohum ve Toprak: Türk Köy Toplumunda Cinsiyet ve Kozmoloji*. İstanbul: İletisim, 2001.

DelVecchio Good, Mary-Jo. "The Medical Imaginary and the Biotechnical Embrace: Subjective Experiences of Clinical Scientists and Patients." In *Subjectivity: Ethnographic Investigations*, ed. João Biehl, Byron Good, and Arthur Kleinman, 362–80. Berkeley: University of California Press, 2007.

Döşemeci, L., M. Yılmaz, M. Cengiz, B. Dora, and A. Ramazanoğlu. "Brain Death and Donor Management in the Intensive Care Unit: Experiences Over the Last Three Years." *Transplantation Proceedings* 36 (2004): 20–21.

Douglas, Mary. *Purity and Danger: An Analysis of the Concepts of Pollution and Taboo*. New York: Routledge, 2000.

Dumit, Joseph. *Picturing Personhood: Brain Scans and Biomedical Identity*. Princeton, N.J.: Princeton University Press, 2004.

Durkheim, Emile. *The Elementary Forms of Religious Life*. Ed. Carol Cosman and Mark Sydney Cladis. New York: Oxford University Press, 2001.

Eliade, Mircae. *The Myth of the Eternal Return, or Cosmos and History*. Princeton, N.J.: Princeton University Press, 1974. First published in 1954.

English Translation of al-Qur'an al-Kerim. Trans. Niyazi Kahveci. Ankara: Akasya, 2007.

Erginer, Gürbüz. *Kurban: Kurbanın Kökenleri ve Anadoluda Kanlı Kurban Ritüelleri*. İstanbul: Yapı Kredi Yayınları, 1997.

Erkol, A. Yılmaz, Hilal Haznedaroğlu, Türkan Özkara, and Hilam Taşkın. "Initiation of Bone and Amnion Banking in Turkey." *Cell and Tissue Banking* no. 2–4 (2003): 169–72.

Farmer, Paul. *Infections and Inequalities: The Modern Plagues*. Berkeley: University of California Press, 1999.

————. *Pathologies of Power: Health, Human Rights and the New War on the Poor*. Berkeley: University of California Press, 2003.

Fassin, Didier. "The Embodiment of Inequality: AIDS as a Social Condition and the Historical Experience in South Africa." Special issue, *EMBO Reports* 4 (2003).

———. *When Bodies Remember: Experiences and Politics of* AIDS *in South Africa.* Berkeley: University of California Press, 2007.

Fischer, Michael M. J. *Anthropological Futures.* Durham, N.C.: Duke University Press, 2009.

———. "Culture and Cultural Analysis as Experimental Systems." *Cultural Anthropology* 22, no. 1 (2007): 1–65.

———. *Emergent Forms of Life and the Anthropological Voice.* Durham, N.C.: Duke University Press, 2003.

———. "Eye(I)ing the Sciences and Their Signifiers (Language, Tropes, Autobiographers): InterViewing for a Cultural Studies of Science and Technology." In *Technoscientific Imaginaries: Conversations, Profiles, and Memoirs,* ed. George Marcus, 43–85. Chicago: University of Chicago Press, 1995.

———. "Four Genealogies for a Recombinant Anthropology of Science and Technology." *Cultural Anthropology* 22, no. 3 (2007): 539–614.

———. *Iran: From Religious Dispute to Revolution.* Cambridge, Mass.: Harvard University Press, 1980.

———. *Mute Dreams, Blind Owls and Dispersed Knowledges: Persian Poesis in the Transnational Circuitry.* Durham, N.C.: Duke University Press, 2004.

Fischer, Michael M. J., and Mehdi Abedi. *Debating Muslims: Cultural Dialogues in Postmodernity and Tradition.* Madison: University of Wisconsin Press, 1990.

Fischer, Michael M. J., and George Marcus. *Anthropology as Cultural Critique: An Experimental Moment in the Human Sciences.* Chicago: University of Chicago Press, 1986.

Fliess, Robert. *The Psychoanalytic Reader: An Anthology of Essential Papers, with Critical Introductions.* New York: International Universities Press, 1948.

Foucault, Michel. *Ethics: Subjectivity and Truth.* Ed. Paul Rabinow. New York: New Press, 1997.

———. "Governmentality." Trans. Rosi Braidotti. In *The Foucault Effect: Studies in Governmentality,* ed. Graham Burchell, Colin Gordon, and Peter Miller, 87–104. Chicago: University of Chicago Press, 1991.

———. *The Order of Things: An Archaeology of the Human Sciences.* New York: Pantheon Books, 1971.

———. *Power/Knowledge: Selected Interviews and Other Writings, 1972–1977.* Ed. Colin Gordon. Brighton: Harvester Press, 1980.

Fox, Renée C., and Judith P. Swazey. *The Courage to Fail: A Social View of Organ Transplants and Dialysis.* New Brunswick, N.J.: Transaction Publishers, 2002.

———. *Spare Parts: Organ Replacement in American Society.* New York: Oxford University Press, 1992.

Freud, Sigmund. *The Interpretation of Dreams.* Trans. Joyce Crick. New York: Oxford University Press, 1999. First published in 1900.

———. *Jokes and Their Relation to the Unconscious.* Trans. James Strachey. New York: Norton, 1989. First published in 1905.

———. "Mourning and Melancholia." In *On Freud's "Mourning and Melancholia."* Ed. Leticia Glocer Fiorini, Thierry Bokanowski, and Sergio Lewkowicz, 19–37. London: The Psychoanalytic Association, 2007. First published in 1915–17.

———. *The Uncanny.* London: Penguin Books, 2003. First published in 1919.

Gadamer, Hans-Georg. *Wahrheit und Methode: Grundzüge einer philosophischen Hermeneutik.* Tübingen: Mohr, 1960.

Galton, Francis. *Inquiries into Human Faculty and Its Development.* London: J. M. Dent and Co., 1908.

Geertz, Clifford. "Common Sense as a Cultural System." In *Local Knowledge: Further Essays in Interpretive Anthropology.* New York: Basic Books, 1983.

———. *The Interpretation of Cultures.* New York: Basic Books, 1973.

Gellner, Ernest. *Postmodernism, Reason and Religion.* New York: Routledge, 1992.

Gennep, Arnold van. *The Rites of Passage.* London: Routledge and Paul, 1960.

Goethe, Johann Wolfgang. *Poetische Werke.* Berlin: Berliner Ausgabe, 1960.

Gökalp, Ziya. *Türk Töresi.* Ankara: Kültür Bakanlığı Yayınları, 1976.

Gökmenoğlu, Hüseyin Tekin. *İslâm'da Şahsiyet Hakları.* Ankara: Türkiye Diyanet Vakfı, 1996.

Göksu, Saime, and Edward Timms. *Romantic Communist: The Life and Work of Nazim Hikmet.* New York: Palgrave Macmillan, 1999.

Gökyay, Orhan Saik. "Dede Korkut Hikayelerinde Şamanlık İzleri." In *Dedem Korkudun Kitabı,* 1010. İstanbul: Kabalcı, 2006.

Göle, Nilüfer. *Modern Mahrem: Medeniyet ve Örtünme.* İstanbul: Metis, 1991.

Grene, David, and Richmond Alexander Lattimore, eds. *The Complete Greek Tragedies—Euripides I.* Chicago: University of Chicago Press, 1955.

"Gündem: Arkadaşsın Ortak Kaderi." *Hürriyet,* April 4, 1998.

"Gündem: Ebru Olayından Sonra Bağış Arttı." *Hürriyet,* November 12, 1997.

"Gündem: Organ Bağışında Büyük Artış Var." *Hürriyet,* January 2, 1998.

Güvenç, Bozkurt. *Türk Kimliği: Kültür tarihinin kaynakları.* Ankara: Kültür Bakanlığı, 2000.

Haberal, Mehmed, ed. "Development of Transplantation in Turkey." *Transplantation Proceedings* 33 (2001): 3027–29.

———. *Doku ve Organ Transplantasyonları.* Ankara: Haberal Eğitim Vakfı, 1993.

Haberal, Mehmed, G. Moray, H. Karakay, Ali, and N. Bilgin. "Transplantation Legislation and Practice in Turkey: A Brief History." *Transplantation Proceedings* 30 (1998): 3644–46.

Haberal, Mehmed, Z. Öner, M. Karamehmetoğlu, H. Gülay, and N. Bilgin. "Cadaver Kidney Transplantation with Cold Ischemia Time from 48 to 95 Hours." *Transplantation Proceedings* 16 (1984): 1330.

Haraway, Donna. *Modest_Witness@Second_Millennium.FemaleMan© _Meets_Onco-Mouse™: Feminism and Technoscience.* New York: Routledge, 1997.

———. *Simians, Cyborgs, and Women: The Reinvention of Nature.* New York: Routledge, 1991.

Hertz, Robert. *Death and the Right Hand.* Glencoe, Ill.: Free Press, 1960.

Hikmet, Nazım. *Beyond the Walls: Selected Poems.* Trans. Ruth Christie, Richard McKane, and Talat Sait Halman. London: Anvil Press Poetry, 2002.

Hill, Brad Jobin. *Hebraica from the Valmadonna Trust.* London: Oxford University Press, 1989.

Hogle, Linda. *Recovering the Nation's Body: Cultural Memory, Medicine and the Politics of Redemption.* New Brunswick, N.J.: Rutgers University Press, 1999.

Hubert, Henri, and Marcel Mauss. *Sacrifice: Its Nature and Function.* Chicago: University of Chicago Press, 1981.

Ilmihal II: Islam ve Toplum. Ankara: Diyanet İşleri Başkanlığı, 2002.

Johnson, Lynt B., Paul C. Kuo, Eugene J. Schweitzer, Lloyd E. Ratner, David K. Klassen, Edward W. Hoehn-Saric, Andrew dela Torre, Matthew R. Weir, Julie Strange, and Stephen T. Bartlett. "Double Renal Allografts Successfully Increase Utilization of Kidneys from Older Donors within a Single Organ Procurement Organization." *Transplantation* 62 (1996): 1581.

Joralemon, Donald. "Organ Wars: The Battle for Body Parts." *Medical Anthropology Quarterly,* n.s., 9, no. 3 (1995): 335–56.

Kahya, E. "Bizde disseksiyon ne zaman ve nasıl başladı?" *Belleten* 172 (1979): 739–59.

Kalyoncu, Güngör Dilmen. *Kurban: Oyun.* İstanbul: Cem Yayınevi, 1979.

Karaman, Hayreddin. "İslam Hukukunda Zaruret Hali." In *İslam'ın Işığında Günün Meseleleri.* İstanbul: İz Yayıncılık, 1992. First published in 1978.

———. *İslam'ın Işığında Günün Meseleleri.* İstanbul: İz Yayıncılık, 2002.

Kardeşoğlu, S. "Batman, The City Where Hope Dies." *Milliyet,* October 19, 2000.

Kazancıgil, Aykut. *XIX. Yüzyılda Osmanlı İmparatorluğunda Anatomi.* Bedizel Zülfikar Şanizade Hayatı ve Eserleri. İstanbul: Özel Yayınlar, 1991.

Kemal, Yaşar. *Tanyeri Horozları.* İstanbul: Adam, 2002.

———. *Yer Demir, Gök Bakır* [Iron earth, copper sky]. İstanbul: Güven Yayınevi, 1963.

Keskioğlu, Osman. *Fıkıh Tarihi ve İslâm Hukuku.* Ankara: Ayyıldız Matbaası, 1969.

Kleinman, Arthur. *Patients and Healers in the Context of Culture: An Exploration of the Borderland between Anthropology, Medicine and Psychiatry.* Berkeley: University of California Press, 1981.

Knorr-Cetina, Karin. *Epistemic Cultures: How the Sciences Make Knowledge.* Cambridge, Mass.: Harvard University Press, 1999.

Küçük, İskender. *Cangüncem, 1984/1993: Günce.* İstanbul: Yapı Kredi Yayınları, 1996.

Küçük, M., M. S. Sever, A. Türkmen, S. Şahin, R. Kazancıoğlu, S. Öztürk, and U. Eldegez. "Demographic Analysis and Outcome Features in a Transplant Outpatient Clinic." *Transplantation Proceedings* 37 (2005): 743–46.

Lacan, Jacques. *Écrits: A Selection.* Trans. Alan Sheridan. New York: Norton, 1977.

———. *The Psychoses,* bk. 3, *The Seminar of Jacques Lacan.* Trans. Russell Gigg, ed. Jacques-Alain Miller. New York: Norton, 1993. First published in 1981.

———. *Speech and Language in Psychoanalysis.* Trans. Anthony Wilden. Baltimore: Johns Hopkins University Press, 1994. First published in 1968.

Landecker, Hannah. *Culturing Life: How Cells Became Technologies.* Cambridge, Mass.: Harvard University Press, 2007.

Lee, Hermione. *Virginia Woolf.* New York: Knopf, 1997.

Lester, David. "Suicide and Islam: Archives of Suicide Research." *International Academy of Suicide Research* 10 (2006): 77–97.

Lévi-Strauss, Claude. *Tristes Tropique.* New York: Penguin, 1992. First published 1955.

Lock, Margaret. *Twice Dead: Organ Transplants and the Reinvention of Death.* Berkeley: University of California Press, 2002.

Lock, Margaret, and Megan Crowley-Matoka. "Organ Transplantation in a Globalized World." Unpublished manuscript. 2007.

Löwith, Karl. *From Hegel to Nietzsche: The Revolution in Nineteenth Century Thought.* New York: Columbia University Press, 1991. First published in 1964.

Lyotard, François. *The Postmodern Condition: A Report on Knowledge.* Trans. Geoff Bennington and Brian Massumi. Minneapolis: University of Minnesota Press, 1984.

Mardin, Şerif. *Din ve Ideoloji.* İstanbul: İletişim Yayınevi, 1983.

Marx, Karl. *Capital: A Critique of Political Economy.* Trans. Ben Fowkes. New York: Penguin Books, 1990. First published in 1867.

Mater, Nadide. *Mehmedin Kitabı: Güneydoğuda Savaşan Askerler Anlatıyor.* İstanbul: Metis, 1998.

Mauss, Marcel. *The Gift: Forms and Functions of Exchange in Archaic Societies.* Translated by W. D. Halls. New York: Routledge, 1990. First published 1924.

Montaigne, Michel de. *The Complete Essays of Montaigne.* Trans. Donald M. Frame. Stanford, Calif.: Stanford University Press, 1965.

Neyzi, Leyla. *İstanbul'da hatırlamak ve unutmak: Birey, Bellek ve Aidiyet.* İstanbul: Tarih Vakfı Yurt Yayınları, 1999.

Nietzsche, Friedrich. *The Birth of Tragedy.* Trans. Douglas Smith. Oxford: Oxford University Press, 2000.

Öner, C. "Beyin Ölümü ve Organ Transplantasyonu." In *Tıbbi Etik Yıllığı* 5. İstanbul, 1996.

Örnek Buken, N. "Organ Aktarımında Beyin Ölümünün Tıbbi, felsefi ve Teolojik Yönleri." *Türkiye Klinikleri Tıp Etiği-Hukuku-Tarihi* 4 (1996): 82–84.

Orwell, George. *1984.* London: Secker and Warburg, 1948.

Özkalıpçı, Gökçen. "Bir Transplantasyon hayali olarak Dabbet-ül Arz," "İ.Ü. İstanbul Tıp fakültesi Transplantasyon Ünitesi," "Ulusal Organ ve Doku Nakli Koordinasyon Sistemi," *Naklen* summer issue (2001).

Pamuk, Orhan. *Snow.* Trans. Maureen Freely. London: Faber and Faber, 2004.

Perico, N., P. Ruggenenti, M. Scalamogna, and G. Remuzzi. "Tackling the Shortage of Donor Kidneys: How to Use the Best That We Have." *American Journal of Nephrology* 23 (2003): 245.

Pessione F., S. Cohen, D. Durand, M. Hourmant, M. Kessler, C. Legendre, G. Mou-
rad, C. Noël, M. N. Peraldi, C. Pouteil-Noble, P. Tuppin, and C. Hiesse. "Multivariate Analysis of Donor Risk Factors for Graft Survival in Kidney Transplantation."
Transplantation 75 (2003): 361.

Peterson, Kristin. "HIV/AIDS and Democracy in Nigeria: Policies, Rights and Thera-
peutic Economies." Ph.D. diss., Rice University, 2004.

Petryna, Adriana. *Life Exposed: Biological Citizens after Chernobyl.* Princeton, N.J.:
Princeton University Press, 2002.

Petryna, Adriana, Andrew Lakoff, and Arthur Kleinman, eds. *Global Pharmaceuticals:
Ethics, Markets, Practices.* Durham, N.C.: Duke University Press, 2007.

Poe, Edgar Allen. "Eleonora." In *The Murders in the Morgue and Other Stories,* 35.
Koeln: Koenemann, 1995. First published in 1842.

Proctor, Robert. *Racial Hygiene: Medicine under the Nazis.* Cambridge, Mass.: Harvard University Press, 1988.

Rabinow, Paul. *Essays on the Anthropology of Reason.* Princeton, N.J.: Princeton
University Press, 1996.

Rheinberger, Hans-Jörg. *Toward a History of Epistemic Things: Synthesizing Proteins in
the Test Tube.* Stanford, Calif.: Stanford University Press, 1997.

Richardson, Ruth. *Death, Dissection and the Destitute.* Chicago: University of Chicago
Press, 2001.

Ricoeur, Paul. *Freud and Philosophy: An Essay on Interpretation.* New Haven, Conn.:
Yale University Press, 1970.

Ritvo, Harriet. *The Platypus and the Mermaid, and Other Figments of the Classifying
Imagination.* Cambridge, Mass.: Harvard University Press, 1997.

Said, Edward W. *Beginnings: Intention and Method.* New York: Basic Books, 1975.

Sanal, Aslıhan. "'Robin Hood' of Techno-Turkey or Organ Trafficking the State of
Ethical Beings." *Culture, Medicine, and Psychiatry* 28, no. 3 (2004): 281–309.

———. "Flesh Mine, Bones Yours." Ph.D. diss., Massachusetts Institute of Technology, 2005.

"Şaşırtan Zihniyet" [Surprising mentality]. *Milliyet,* June 23, 1999.

Scheper-Hughes, Nancy. "The Global Traffic in Human Organs." *Current Anthropology* 41, no. 2 (2000): 191–224.

———. "Parts Unknown: Undercover Ethnography of the Organs-trafficking Underworld." *Ethnography* 5, no. 1 (2004): 29–73.

———. "Rotten Trade: Millennial Capitalism, Human Values and Global Justice in
Organs Trafficking." *Journal of Human Rights* 2, no. 2 (2003): 197–226.

Scheper-Hughes, Nancy, and Loïc Wacquant, eds. *Commodifying Bodies.* Thousand
Oaks, Calif.: Sage Publications, 2002.

Schimmel, Annemarie. *Tanrının Yeryüzündeki İşaretleri.* İstanbul: Kabalcı Yayınevi,
2004.

Şehirli, Ümit Süleyman, E. Saka, and C. Sarıkaya. "Attitudes of Turkish Anatomists
toward Cadaver Donation." *Clinical Anatomy* 17 (2004): 677–81.

Şen, F. "The Truth Behind the Suicides." *Sabah*, September 16, 2000.

Şener, Cemal. *Alevi Törenleri: Abdal Musa, Veli Baba Sultan, Hamza Baba, Hacı Bektaş Veli*. İstanbul: Ant Yayınları, 1991.

Sever, Aysan, and Rüstem Erkan. "The Dark Faces of Poverty, Patriarchal Oppression, and Social Change: Female Suicides in Batman, Turkey." Working Paper #282, Office of Women in International Development, Michigan State University, 2004.

Sharp, Lesley. *Bodies, Commodities, and Biotechnologies: Death, Mourning, and Scientific Desire in the Realms of Human Organ Transfer*. New York: Columbia University Press, 2007.

———. "The Commodification of the Body and Its Parts." *Annual Review of Anthropology* 29 (2000): 287–328.

———. "Organ Transplantation as a Transformative Experience: Anthropological Insights into the Restructuring of the Self." *Medical Anthropology Quarterly* 9, no. 3 (1995): 357–89.

Simmel, Georg. *Das Individuelle Gesetz: Philosophische Exkurse*. Ed. and trans. Michael Landmann. Frankfurt am Main: Suhrkamp, 1968.

Smith, Jane I., and Yvonne Yazbeck Haddad. *The Islamic Understanding of Death and Resurrection*. Albany: State University of New York Press, 1981.

Steward, Sue. "Waxing Lyrical on the Fragile Body." *London Evening Standard*, March 7, 2005, 75.

Sunder-Rajan, Kaushik. *Biocapital: The Constitution of Postgenomic Life*. Durham, N.C.: Duke University Press, 2006.

Susser, E., M. T. Finnerty, and N. Sohler. "Acute Psychoses: A Proposed Diagnosis for ICD-11 and DSM-V." *Psychiatric Quarterly* 67, no. 3 (1996): 165–76.

Tabakoğlu, A., I. Kutluer, I. Kara, I. Özel, A. Davudoglu, M. Özel, and A. Kara. *Bilgi-Bilim ve İslam II: Tartısmalı İlmi Toplantılar Dizisi*. İstanbul: İlmi Neşriyat A.S., 1992.

Tanpınar, Ahmet Hamdi. *Saatleri Ayarlama Enstitüsü*. İstanbul: Dergah Yayınları, 1962.

Taşdemir, A., and S. Genç. "Çıldırtan Ayrılık." *Hürriyet*, November 7, 1997.

Taussig, Michael. *Shamanism, Colonialism, and the Wild Man: A Study in Terror and Healing*. Chicago: University of Chicago Press, 1987.

Tavaslı, Yusuf. *Tam Dua Kitabı*. İstanbul: Tavaslı Yayınları, N.d.

T.C Basbakanlik Aile Arastirma Kurumu [Turkish Republic: Family Research Institution]. *Aile içi şiddetin sebep ve sonuçları* [The causes and consequences of Inter-family violence]. Ankara, 1995.

Temizyürek, M., E. Özgümüş, A. Altas, H. Erdoğan, N. Gökçe, B. Özgürbüz, and S. Akyel. *Basinda Transplantasyonun 20 Yılı*. Ankara: Haberal Egitim Vakfı, 1996.

Titiz, İzzet. *Renal Transplantasyona Pratik Yaklaşım*. İstanbul: Eczacıbaşı İlaç Pazarlama, 2000.

"Türkiyede Organ Nakli Sorunları ve Çözüm Yolları Paneli 2." *Bir Yudum Sağlık* 1, no. 2 (May 2, 2006).

Turkle, Sherry. *Evocative Objects*. Cambridge, Mass.: MIT Press, 2007.

———. *The Inner History of Devices*. Cambridge, Mass.: MIT Press, 2008.

———. *Life on the Screen: Identity in the Age of the Internet*. New York: Simon and Schuster, 1997.

———. *The Second Self: Computers and the Human Spirit*. New York: Simon and Schuster, 1984.

Turner, Victor W. *The Ritual Process: Structure and Anti-structure*. New York: Aldine de Gruyter, 1995.

Unat, Ekrem Kadri. *Dünyada ve Türkiye'de 1850 yılından sonra Tıp Dallarında İlerlemenin Tarihi*. İstanbul: Cerrahpaşa Tıp Fakültesi Vakfı Yayınları, 1988.

Veli, Orhan. "Kitabe-I Seng-I Mezar III." In *Orhan Veli: Bütün Şiirleri*. İstanbul: YKY, 2003.

Weber, Max. *The Protestant Ethic and the Spirit of Capitalism*. Chicago: Roxburry, 2001. First published in 1904.

White, Jenny B. *Islamist Mobilization in Turkey: A Study in Venacular Politics*. Seattle: University of Washington Press, 2002.

Wijdicks, E. "Brain Death Worldwide: Accepted Fact but No Global Consensus in Diagnostic Criteria." *Neurology* 58 (January 2002): 2.

Woolf, Virginia. *To the Lighthouse*. New York: Knopf, 1991. First published in 1927.

"Yardımı kibarca reddettik" [We gently refused the aid]. *Sabah Online*, August 22, 1999.

Yayla, A. 2005. "Özal Reformları ve Liberalizm." In *Modern Türkiyede Siyasi Düşünce*, vol. 7, *Liberalizm*, 587. İstanbul: İletişim, 2005.

Yılmaz, Aybige. "Victims, Villains and Guardian Angels: Batman Suicide Stories." *Westminster Papers in Communication and Culture* 1, no. 1 (2004): 66–92.

Zaehner, R. C. *Mysticism, Sacred and Profane: An Inquiry into Some Varieties of Praeternatural Experience*. Oxford: Clarendon Press, 1957.

Zeydan, Abdülkerim. "Halat-ud-Darure Fi's-Şeriat'il-İslamiyye." *Bagdat Journal of Islamic Studies* 3 (1970): 5–72. Translated into Turkish in 1978 by Hayrettin Karaman in *İslamın Işığında Günün Meseleleri*, 171–265. İstanbul: İz Yayıncılık, 2002.

Zweig, Stefan. *Baumeister der Welt: Balzac, Dickens, Dostojewski, Hèolderlin, Kleist, Nietzsche, Casanova, Stendhal, Tolstoi*. Frankfurt am Main: S. Fischer, 1951.

FILMS AND TELEVISION SHOWS

All About My Mother [*Todo Sobre de Mi Madre*]. Dir. Pedro Almodóvar. Hollywood: Sony Pictures Classics, 1999.

Arena Team. Dir. Uğur Dündar. Channel D (İstanbul). February 20, 1997.

———. Dir. Uğur Dündar. Channel D (İstanbul). December 14, 1999.

———. Dir. Uğur Dündar. Channel D (İstanbul). February 2000.

CNN Türk. "Sağlık Dünya Böbrek Günü." Television interview with Dr. Arıcı of Hacettepe University, March 2, 2007.

Kurtlar Vadisi [The valley of the wolves]. Television series. Dir. Serdar Akar, Mustafa Sevki Doğan, and Osman Sinav. İstanbul: Pana Film, 2003–5.

Kurtlar Vadisi—Irak [The valley of the wolves—Iraq]. Film. Dir. Serdar Akar and Sadullah Sentürk. İstanbul: Pana Film, 2006.

Metropolis. Film. Dir. Fritz Lang. Hollywood: Paramount Pictures, 1927.

NTV News. Television interview with Alper Demirbaş, Akdeniz University, May 5, 2007.

INDEX

ASLIHAN SANAL is a cultural anthropologist who focuses on science and medical technology. She received her Ph.D. from MIT in 2005 and is currently working as an independent scholar in Germany. This is her first book.

Library of Congress Cataloging-in-Publication Data

Sanal, Aslıhan, 1971–
New organs within us : transplants and the moral economy / Aslihan Sanal.
p. cm. — (Experimental futures)
Includes bibliographical references and index.
ISBN 978-0-8223-4889-4 (cloth : alk. paper)
ISBN 978-0-8223-4912-9 (pbk. : alk. paper)
1. Kidneys—Transplantation—Patients—Turkey. 2. Transplantation of organs, tissues, etc.—Turkey. 3. Transplantation of organs, tissues, etc.—Moral and ethical aspects. 4. Organ trafficking—Turkey.
I. Title. II. Series: Experimental futures.
RD575.S263 2011
617.4'61059209561—dc22   2010044957